Chart your weekly *Get Fit* progress as you gradually achieve your goals. This is a great way to stay motivated to continu⋯ ⋯ ⋯ ⋯ fitness⋯

WEEKLY RESULTS

	Weight	Fat%	BMI					BP
WEEK 1								
WEEK 2								
WEEK 3								
WEEK 4								
WEEK 5								
WEEK 6								
WEEK 7								
WEEK 8								
WEEK 9								
WEEK 10								

FITNESS PROGRESS CHART

Weekly Weight Chart

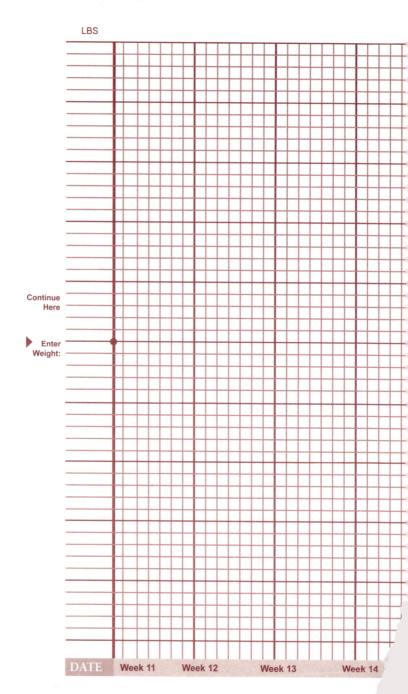

LBS

Continue Here

▶ Enter Weight:

| DATE | Week 11 | Week 12 | Week 13 | Week 14 |

I Will
GET FIT
This Time!

WORKOUT JOURNAL

Includes

HELPFUL DAILY TIPS

to GET FIT!

Alex A. Lluch

I WILL GET FIT THIS TIME WORKOUT JOURNAL

BY ALEX A. LLUCH

Nutritional and fitness guidelines based on information provided by the United States Food and Drug Administration, Food and Nutrition Information Center, National Agricultural Library, Agricultural Research Service, and the U.S. Department of Agriculture.

Photo Credits:
Cover (from left to right, top to bottom): © Moodboard/Corbis, © Jamie Grill/Corbis, © Charles Gullung/Zefa/Corbis, © Amana Productions Inc./Getty Images

ISBN-13: 978-1-887169-97-4

Printed in China

TABLE OF CONTENTS

TABLE OF CONTENTS

TABLE OF CONTENTS

INTRODUCTION

Getting fit will help you live a long, healthy, and enjoyable life. You don't have to live at the gym or make radical changes in your lifestyle. The benefits of getting fit are many, such as physical well-being, reduced stress, better sleep, increased self-esteem and greater self-confidence. With a combination of regular exercise and sensible eating, you will feel stronger, have greater endurance, and more energy.

It is true that becoming fit will involve commitment on your part. You will need to set aside some time each day to improve your physical conditioning and make healthy eating a priority. By reading this book you will find that getting fit can be fun and enjoyable. You will find by using the information contained in this book, getting fit is easier than you think.

WHAT IS THIS BOOK ABOUT?

This book will guide you through the basic principles of fitness and then teach you how to integrate them into your daily life. By encouraging you to examine your current fitness level and identify your personal goals, this book will help you create a personalized workout routine that you will follow and even enjoy.

This book is not a list of instructions that must be followed to the letter, but rather information and a journal that will accompany you on your journey to a new and healthier you. There are no get-fit-quick remedies in these pages. Instead, you will find real information that will help you make lasting changes to your lifestyle. Using the journal, you will plan your exercise routine and record your successes as you work toward a healthier and more satisfying lifestyle.

The pages that follow will also help you change the way you think about fitness. This book throws out the "no pain, no gain" and "do-or-die" attitudes and teaches you to view getting fit as a process that should be enjoyed. It will help you shift away from unrealistic media-driven expectations regarding fitness. This book will encourage you to adopt a more personal view of fitness that is based primarily on the effort you put forth. You will also discover how your success in getting fit will spill over into all aspects of your life.

WHO SHOULD READ THIS BOOK?

This book is for anyone who wants to learn how to get and stay fit. No matter what your age, this book will show you how anyone can improve their quality of life by adding regular physical exercise to their daily routine.

Parents should read this book, not only for themselves, but to be a good models for their children. Your children look up to you and learn from your actions. By showing them that fitness is an important aspect of your life, you will teach them to respect their own bodies and to make the right choices to stay fit and healthy.

WHAT IS IN THIS BOOK?

This book is divided into seven parts and a fitness journal. Each part focuses on a specific aspect of physical fitness. They are arranged in a linear progression from baseline evaluation to creating your own personalized fitness routine.

Part 1: Understanding Fitness, reviews the benefits of adding a fitness routine to your life and provides simple methods for you to comprehensively evaluate your current fitness level. This section will help you identify realistic fitness goals and develop a plan to achieve these goals.

Part 2: Components of a Complete Workout Program, focuses on the specific components of a complete exercise program: cardiovascular, strength and flexibility training. It shows how, individually and together, these three components will optimize your ability to perform physically. You will come away with a new understanding of how these types of exercises can work to transform your body.

Part 3: Things You Should Know about Nutrition, evaluates the role of nutrition in your physical health. You will learn how the foods you eat affect your physical performance and how proper nutrition can dramatically improve fitness.

Part 4: Optimizing Your Diet to Maximize Your Results, examines how to use food to maximize results and reach your personal goal. By dispelling old myths about diet and nutrition, you will discover the keys to creating a diet that helps you lose weight, gain muscle mass, and increase energy levels. You will also learn the importance of drinking water and how proper hydration plays a key role in your physical fitness. You will learn proper hydration techniques and come away with a new understanding of how water plays a pivotal role in determining your fitness level.

Part 5: Work Out Products and Services, discusses other factors that are related to fitness, such as how to choose the right methods and venues for exercise. The advantages and disadvantages of gym memberships, home workouts, and personal trainers will be examined.

Part 6: Personal Data, provides a series of worksheets and tables to help you develop your own fitness goals and track your progress towards these goals. This section is designed to get you motivated and to keep you motivated throughout your fitness program.

Part 7: Daily Workout Journal, is where you can keep a detailed record of your daily workouts. You can note your daily goals, your weight, the exercises you completed, and your results. Every page has space available for you to make comments regarding your progress toward your goals.

This book presents a fresh perspective on health and fitness. It is designed to give you the tools to get fit and help you maintain your motivation throughout the process. Finally, the book will give you all the confidence you'll need to achieve your fitness goals.

OTHER GREAT FEATURES OF THIS WORKOUT JOURNAL

"Away from Home" Workout Journal: Take this handy, pocket-sized journal with you to the gym to help you keep track of your workouts. This mini-journal provides space in which you can record cardio, strength, flexibility, and group exercises that you complete each day. It also allows you to keep track of your food and water intake, as well as monitor your progress.

Workout Progress Charts: These charts will allow you to keep track of your progress. You can record your measurements, evaluate your results, and then set new goals as your fitness levels improve.

"I Did It!" Stickers: Self-adhesive stars can be peeled off and placed in the journal each day as you achieve your daily goal.

Nutritional Facts on Popular Food Items: This comprehensive list provides nutrition values for hundreds of foods so that you can plan a diet that will help you reach your fitness goals.

PART 1: UNDERSTANDING FITNESS

So you've decided to take some positive steps toward improving your fitness. Congratulations! Even before you head for your first workout, consider why fitness is important to you. This will help you set goals and stay motivated. It's also important to think about your current fitness level. Knowing your starting point will help you set realistic goals and move safely toward achieving those goals. Finally, think about how you'll achieve your goals. The first three chapters of this book aim to help you find the answers to these questions.

REASONS FOR GETTING AND STAYING FIT

What motivates people to get and stay fit? Why should people spend time, money and energy working out and being physically active when today's society is filled with more responsibilities and less time to accomplish them than ever before?

It's no surprise that over 60 percent of adults in the U.S. do not get the recommended amount of daily physical activity. Our long work hours, advances in modern technology, and increasing demands of our daily lives have led to a more sedentary lifestyle. In addition, the rise of fast food consumption and the availability of convenience foods have caused us to develop unhealthy eating habits. Our demanding work schedules, poor fitness and dietary habits have led Americans to become among the most obese and stressed people in the world.

In the past you may have not fully understood the benefits of daily physical activity or the consequences of a sedentary lifestyle. Or you may not have been able to overcome the obstacles that prevented you from working out. Maybe you did not know how to establish good habits that would enable you to stick with a physical fitness program. This time, with the information provided in this book combined with your commitment, you will get fit, feel great and enjoy a better quality of life.

Fitness is a choice you can make. You can decide to take the stairs versus the elevator, go to the gym instead of watching television, and wake up early and go for a run instead of sleeping in. Since you have purchased this book, you have probably already chosen to improve your physical fitness. You most likely have your own reasons for making that choice. You may have decided that you want to fit into a new pair of jeans; perhaps you've decided to run a marathon and need to get in shape; or maybe you've simply decided to lead a healthier lifestyle. Regardless of your motives, there are many valid and scientifically proven benefits of working out.

HEALTH BENEFITS

Research regarding the relationship between fitness and health is extensive and has been ongoing for decades. The results are clear: You will live longer if you are physically active. A Surgeon General's report on the benefits of physical activity concludes that even moderate exercise can substantially reduce the risk of developing or dying from diabetes, colon cancer and obesity-related illnesses.

Not being physically active can actually increase your risk of certain diseases. People who don't exercise are almost twice as likely to develop heart disease, which is the leading cause of death in the U.S.. Health experts say that millions of individuals in America suffer from many other chronic diseases that can be prevented through exercise. Clearly, it is in your best interest to be physically active.

Participating in a daily workout routine can benefit your health, just as inactivity can harm it. Scientific research conclusively proves that exercise helps lower cholesterol, reduce blood pressure, and prevent osteoporosis. Ongoing research is also providing evidence that exercise also protects against arthritis, certain kinds of cancer, and numerous other diseases.

PHYSICAL BENEFITS

The physical effects of exercise can be extremely gratifying. There are three main benefits that you will experience when you incorporate a workout into your daily routine. First, you will experience an overall improvement in your physical appearance as you increase lean muscle mass, lose weight, and gain strength. Second, you will benefit from an increased metabolism as your body becomes .more efficient at burning food for energy. In addition, you will feel more rested and have more energy because you will experience improved sleep.

How exercise achieves these benefits is not mysterious. For example, a daily exercise program can help you look better by allowing you to control your weight and build muscle mass. Without exercise, muscle mass decreases and body fat increases. When you work out on a regular basis, the body becomes more defined, toned and athletic. The process of gaining muscle mass occurs when a muscle is repeatedly activated against some form of resistance, such as when you lift weights. In response to this exertion, a muscle will grow larger and stronger in order to fulfill this new physical demand.

Increasing your lean muscle mass actually increases your ability to burn fat. Muscles consume more calories than other types of tissues do. You can burn approximately 50 more calories a day for every pound of added muscle. A regular workout routine, combined with a sensible diet, allows the body to use more calories than it is ingesting. This forces the body to convert stored fat into energy. Body weight decreases and you become stronger, leaner, and more defined. Clothes fit better. You stand taller and straighter, since stronger muscles help improve your posture; overall you look and feel more confident.

One of the many physical benefits of exercise is an improved metabolism. Metabolism refers to the amount of calories your body burns to stay alive. Specifically, it refers to the speed and efficiency with which the body is able to break down food and convert it into energy. Regular exercise helps facilitate the body's ability to burn calories by maximizing the flow of oxygen-laden blood throughout the body. The more oxygen your body receives, the more calories you burn.

Regular exercise is one way to foster healthy sleep. The body has a natural cycle in which it alternates between states of inactivity during sleep and arousal while awake. These cycles are symbiotic, meaning that they depend on one another. If the body remains too sedentary during its active phase, it may have a difficult transition into its sleep phase. However, if the body is forced to work and intensify its active period, it will conversely enter into a deeper rest period. Tests have shown that those who maintain a regular exercise routine benefit from a more consistent and restful sleep. Increased sleep results in an improvement in vitality, mental acuity and mood.

PSYCHOLOGICAL BENEFITS

The psychological improvements that result through regular exercise are just as abundant and transforming as the health and physical benefits. Evidence shows that those who exercise moderately on a regular basis have lower levels of anxiety and are less likely to suffer from depression. Routine exercisers also report increased self-esteem and overall happiness. These feelings are most intense for a few hours after exercise due to the release of naturally occurring substances, called endorphins, into the bloodstream. Endorphins relax muscles and give a person an overall feeling of relaxation and contentment. Research suggests that as the body increases its ability to exercise it also increases its ability to produce endorphins. Consequently, more exercise leads to feeling better longer.

Maintaining a fitness routine creates a feeling of accomplishment and confidence. Many people find that success in transforming themselves physically has a collateral effect in other aspects of their lives. For example, increased confidence and self-esteem can enhance your ability in your professional and social life.

ADDITIONAL BENEFITS OF PHYSICAL ACTIVITY

The combined health, physical and psychological benefits of physical fitness foster an overall lifestyle change. With increased energy and self-confidence, new opportunities are opened. Whereas a sedentary lifestyle is limiting, a healthy, fit lifestyle expands your horizons. Many people find that increased self-confidence and energy can lead to an increased desire to engage in new social and physical activities. The end result is an improvement in one's overall quality of life.

People who maintain a regular physical fitness routine find an increased desire to engage in new physical activities. Simply put, bodies in motion are more likely to remain in motion. Increased energy allows individuals to pursue new activities that were hindered by their previous sedentary lifestyle. People who maintain a regular fitness routine are more able to pursue activities that they find personally satisfying. For example, those who enjoy nature have renewed energy to take hikes and bicycle rides. Those who enjoy sports are able to play and compete at a more competitive level.

A healthy, active lifestyle increases opportunities for people to make new friends. Exercise itself may become the source of social interactions. Whether in the form of casual conversation with others in the gym or by joining an organized class, exercise is an excellent way to make friends or develop new interests. While classic forms of exercise like team sports and spinning (bicycling) classes continue to be popular, alternative forms like ballroom dancing and yoga have also gained new interest and availability.

YOUR CURRENT FITNESS LEVEL

Each individual has his or her unique potential for physical fitness based on the interaction of genetics, health status and lifestyle. Therefore, the first step in getting fit is determining your current physical condition. This information will be used to establish your baseline level of fitness. This chapter contains a series of simple tests used to quantify your starting point on the road to fitness. These tests will focus on cardiovascular health, body composition, strength and flexibility. The information provided in this section can be used as a guide to systematically tailor an exercise plan to reach your personal fitness goals.

Record the results of these tests on the Fitness Test Results Worksheet on page 27. In later chapters, these numbers will be used to prepare realistic fitness goals and track personal progress and success.

IMPORTANT REMINDER: A doctor should be consulted before beginning any rigorous exercise program. This is especially important if you are taking medication for high blood pressure or are being treated for any other physical condition.

ASSESSING YOUR CURRENT FITNESS LEVEL

Begin by assessing your current fitness level. Use this assessment to create a realistic fitness plan. This baseline assessment includes attention to (1) heart rate, (2) blood pressure, (3) body composition, (4) strength, and (5) flexibility.

HEART RATE

The heart rate is a leading indicator of your baseline fitness level and can be used as a guide to maximize the results of cardiovascular exercise. The heart is a specialized muscle that is designed to pump the blood needed to maintain all of your bodily functions. Blood brings oxygen and nutrients to every part of the body. A heart's performance is essential to sustaining life all the way down to the cellular level.

Your heart rate is the number of times your heart beats in a minute. This number is a clear indicator of the strength of your heart. A strong heart pumps more effectively with each contraction and therefore doesn't need to beat as fast to supply the body with blood. A high heart rate indicates that the heart is not as efficient at circulating blood and therefore needs to pump faster to keep up with your body's needs. As your heart becomes better at pumping blood through regular exercise, you will find that your heart rate will decrease. Find your resting and active heart rates by following the simple instructions below. Use these numbers to determine your current fitness level.

A resting heart rate is simply the number of times the heart beats in a minute when you're not moving around. It is important that you sit or lie down and remain motionless for at least two minutes before making this measurement. Once you're completely relaxed, place two fingers against the inside of the wrist or alongside the neck. Count the number of beats for fifteen seconds and then multiply that number by four. Record this figure in the Fitness Test Results Worksheet on page 27. Compare your heart rate to the table, which provides heart rate fitness levels by age and gender.

Resting Heart Rate Fitness by Age and Gender

MEN BY AGE GROUP							
Age		18–25	26–35	36–45	46–55	56–65	65+
Excellent	Resting Heart Rate	50–60	50–61	51–62	51–63	52–61	51–61
Good		61–68	62–69	63–69	64–70	62–70	62–68
Average		69–76	70–77	70–78	71–79	71–78	69–75
Fair		77–80	78–80	79–81	80–83	79–80	76–78
Poor		81+	81+	82+	84+	81+	79+

WOMEN BY AGE GROUP							
Age		18–25	26–35	36–45	46–55	56–65	65+
Excellent	Resting Heart Rate	55–64	55–63	55–63	55–64	55–63	55–63
Good		65–72	64–71	64–72	65–72	64–72	64–71
Average		73–80	72–78	73–80	73–79	73–79	72–79
Fair		81-83	79-81	81-83	80-82	80-82	80-81
Poor		84+	82+	84+	83+	83+	82+

Fitness can also be evaluated in terms of what is called your active heart rate. An active heart rate indicates your heart's maximum potential or ability to work under strain. An active heart rate is important for measuring improvement in your fitness, specifically with regard to aerobic fitness.

BLOOD PRESSURE

It is important to determine your blood pressure before starting a physical fitness program. Those suffering from high blood pressure should contact a medical professional before beginning any physical fitness routine. Blood pressure is the force of blood against the arteries and is created by the heart as it pumps blood through the circulatory system. Like all muscles, the heart cycles between contracting and relaxing; blood pressure varies accordingly. Systolic blood pressure refers to the pressure when the heart contracts. Diastolic pressure refers to the pressure when the heart relaxes. Blood pressure is expressed by these two figures, with the systolic reading listed over the diastolic figure (e.g., 130/90).

Many pharmacies are equipped with machines that allow customers to measure their own blood pressure. This may serve as a quick way to generally measure baseline blood pressure, but a trained professional can give you the most reliable reading. When you're visiting your doctor in advance of beginning an exercise program, your blood pressure will certainly be checked and recorded. Write your blood pressure on the Fitness Test Results Worksheet on page 27. Compare your blood pressure to the table on the following page, which lists blood pressure figures and their corresponding risk categories.

Individuals who are overweight often suffer from high blood pressure, or hypertension. Hypertension is dangerous because it strains the heart as it pumps blood through the body. Over time, the strain can lead to heart muscle breakdown and deterioration. This leaves the heart weakened and increases the chance of a heart attack, stroke, and heart failure. In addition, hypertension can lead to chronic kidney failure.

BODY COMPOSITION

The body functions best when it consists of a proper proportion of muscle, fat, organs and bone. Your body composition is determined by the ratio of these elements against the body's mass. While bone and organs' mass and weight remain relatively constant, everyone's fat and muscle weight

Blood Pressure and Corresponding Risk Level

Systolic	Diastolic	Stage and Health Risk
210	120	High Blood Pressure • Hypertension Stage 4 • Very Severe Risk
180	110	High Blood Pressure • Hypertension Stage 3 • Severe
160	100	High Blood Pressure • Hypertension Stage 2 • Moderate Risk
140	90	High Blood Pressure • Hypertension Stage 1 • Mild Risk
140	90	Borderline High
130	90	High Normal
120	85	Normal • Optimum
110	75	Low Normal
90	60	Borderline Low
60	40	Low Blood Pressure • Hypotension
50	33	Very Low Blood Pressure • Extreme Danger

varies. The percent of body weight that is made up of fat and muscle is an important indicator of body composition and overall fitness. Without proper amounts of both muscle and fat, the body will fail to work at its optimum level.

A person who appears thin may still have a high fat percentage and therefore be unhealthy. People who undergo crash or extreme diets will often lose more muscle mass than fat. If you try to lose weight by dieting without exercising, lean muscle mass may decrease, resulting in an increased fat percentage. Exercise will keep that from happening. Regular exercise forces muscles to engage and work to exhaustion. This, coupled with adequate rest, forces your muscles to adapt by growing larger and stronger. The increased muscle mass diminishes your body's fat percentage and increases its overall health.

Fat is essential to many functions of the body. However, excess fat, especially in the waist area, puts you at increased risk of cardiovascular disease and other health problems such as heart attacks, strokes, and diabetes. In addition, new research shows a correlation between most forms of cancer (except skin cancer) and excess body fat. While genetic predispositions and environmental factors can put you at risk of developing cancer and many other diseases, excess weight increases these risks by making it more difficult for the body to fight off infection and rebuild damaged tissues.

Body composition and fat percentages can be determined in numerous ways:

Hydrostatic Weighing: The most accurate method of measuring body composition is called hydrostatic weighing. This involves weighing a person in air and then again while submerged in water. However accurate this method might be, it is not very practical due to the specialized equipment needed and the complexity of the procedure.

Bioelectrical Impedance Analysis (BIA): The BIA is a computerized examination that helps medical professionals determine the specific composition of the body, including its fat percentage. This is a non-invasive test administered by a doctor and takes about ten minutes. A BIA can also detect the presence of disease, nutrient and water deficiency, environmental and industrial pollutants, oxidative damage and other ailments. With this information a health care provider can create a fitness and diet routine that helps correct a variety of conditions.

Caliper Test: The most common and relatively accurate method for measuring body fat is what's known as a skin fold, or caliper, test. Using a specialized instrument called a caliper, the person conducting the test pinches folds of skin on various locations throughout the body. This test is available at many gyms or fitness facilities.

Body Mass Index (BMI): Less accurate than hydrostatic weighing or a caliper skin fold test, the BMI uses a person's height and weight to determine an approximate fat percentage. Healthcare professionals often use a person's BMI to determine his or her cardiovascular health risk. While all bodies are different, they all generally conform to this scale. While each person's frame varies, the range provided in the BMI takes that into consideration. Your BMI can be determined by taking your weight (in kilograms) and dividing it by its height (in meters) squared; the formula is simple: $Kg/m2$ = BMI. Your approximate BMI can be found using your body's height (feet) and weight (lbs) in the following table. This table also shows the cardiovascular risks associated with various ranges of BMI readings.

Body Mass Index and Cardiovascular Risk Chart for Men and Women

BMI	19	20	21	22	23	24	25	26	27	28	29	30	31	32	33	34	35
Height							**weight in pounds**										
4'10"	91	96	100	105	110	115	119	124	129	134	138	143	148	153	158	162	167
4'11"	94	99	104	109	114	119	124	128	133	138	143	148	153	158	163	168	173
5'	97	102	107	112	118	123	128	133	138	143	148	153	158	163	158	174	179
5'1"	100	106	111	116	122	127	132	137	143	148	153	158	164	169	174	180	185
5'2"	104	109	115	120	126	131	136	142	147	153	158	164	169	175	180	186	191
5'3"	107	113	118	124	130	135	141	146	152	158	163	169	175	180	186	191	197
5'4"	110	116	122	128	134	140	145	151	157	163	169	174	180	186	192	197	204
5'5"	114	120	126	132	138	144	150	156	162	168	174	180	186	192	198	204	210
5'6"	118	124	130	136	142	148	155	161	167	173	179	186	192	198	204	210	216
5'7"	121	127	134	140	146	153	159	166	172	178	185	191	198	204	211	217	223
5'8"	125	131	138	144	151	158	164	171	177	184	190	197	203	210	216	223	230
5'9"	128	135	142	149	155	162	169	176	182	189	196	203	209	216	223	230	236
5'10"	132	139	146	153	160	167	174	181	188	195	202	209	216	222	229	236	243
5'11"	136	143	150	157	165	172	179	186	193	200	208	215	222	229	236	243	250
6'	140	147	154	162	169	177	184	191	199	206	213	221	228	235	242	250	258
6'1"	144	151	159	166	174	182	189	197	204	212	219	227	235	242	250	257	265
6'2"	148	155	163	171	179	186	194	202	210	218	225	233	241	249	256	264	272
6'3"	152	160	168	176	184	192	200	208	216	224	232	240	248	256	264	272	279
	Healthy						**Overweight**					**Obese**					

Record your approximate BMI on the Fitness Test Results Worksheet on page 27.

STRENGTH

Your body's physical strength shows the condition of your muscles and their ability to function at maximum output. Strength is the amount of force a muscle can produce. It can be measured in the amount of weight the muscle can lift or how much force it can exert as you jump, hit a golf ball, or engage in other activities. By measuring your muscles' strength you can get a sense of your overall fitness. This measurement can help you create a fitness plan and measure future successes. Follow the instructions for each of the following strength tests and record the results in the Fitness Results Worksheet on page 27.

Push-up Test: This test focuses on the strength and endurance of muscles in your upper body. Gently stretch and warm up your arm, chest and shoulder muscles. Avoid over-exertion in order to get the most accurate test results. Men should assume the traditional push-up position, with only the hands and tips of the toes touching the ground. Women should assume the bent knee position, with knees and hands touching the ground. No matter which position you use, you should keep the head, neck and back aligned. Start by bending your arms and slowly lowering your chest until it's four inches from the ground, keeping your back and legs straight. Then straighten the arms and push your body back into the starting position. Be sure not to lock your elbows. The back and legs should remain straight and the head and neck in line at all times. Repeat this as many times as you can while maintaining proper form. Count the number of repetitions before fatigue forces you to stop.

Record the number in the Fitness Test Results Worksheet on page 27. The following table will help you estimate your condition based on your age, gender, and the number of push-ups you can do.

Push-up Fitness for Men

Men's Age		13-19	20's	30's	40's	50's	60's
Excellent		45+	40+	35+	29+	25+	23+
Good	No. of Push-ups	31-41	26-35	22-29	18-25	15-22	14-20
Average		26-29	22-25	18-21	15-17	12-14	10-13
Fair		14-24	12-21	9-17	7-14	5-11	3-9
Poor		14 or less	12 or less	9 or less	7 or less	5 or less	3 or less

Push-up Fitness for Women

Women's Age	13-19	20's	30's	40's	50's	60's
Excellent	32+	30+	28+	24+	20+	18+
Good	21–28	19–26	18–26	15–22	12–18	11–16
Average	17–20	16–18	14–17	12–14	10–12	8–10
Fair	9–16	8–15	5–13	4–11	3–9	2–7
Poor	8-	7-	4-	3-	2-	1-

(No. of Push-ups)

Sit up-Test: The sit-up test assesses your abdominal muscles' fitness and stamina. Lie on the floor, facing up with knees bent and place your feet shoulder-width apart. Start by pressing your lower back into the ground and place your arms across your chest. Lift your head, neck and shoulders off the floor and bring your body into a sitting position by engaging the stomach muscles. The abdomen should be contracted as your upper body is brought to a 90-degree angle with the floor. Then slowly roll back down into the starting position while keeping the abdominal muscles tight.

Record the number of repetitions per minute in the Fitness Test Results Worksheet on page 27 and compare your number with the following chart.

One Minute Sit-up Test for Men

Men's Age	18–25	26–35	36–45	46–55	56–65	65+
Excellent	49+	46+	42+	36+	32+	29+
Good	41–48	39–45	34–41	27–35	23–31	20–28
Average	34–40	31–38	25–33	21–26	16–22	14–19
Fair	30–33	29–30	22–24	18–20	14–15	11–13
Poor	29-	28-	21-	17-	13-	10-

(No. of Sit-ups)

One Minute Sit-up Test for Women

Women's Age		18–25	26–35	36–45	46–55	56–65	65+
Excellent		43+	39+	33+	27 +	24+	23+
Good	No. of Sit-ups	35–42	31–38	25–32	20–26	16–23	15–22
Average		28–34	24–30	18–24	13–19	9–15	10–14
Fair		23–27	19–23	14–17	9–12	6–8	4–9
Poor		22-	18-	13-	8-	5-	3-

Squat Test: The Squat test focuses on the strength of the lower body. Stand up straight with your feet shoulder-width apart. Just as if you are sitting back into a chair, bring your hips back and lower your body until your upper legs are parallel to the floor. Keep your knees and heels aligned at all times. With your head and chest lifted, return to a standing position. A chair may be placed underneath as a guide, but must not be used to rest in between squats. Count how many squats are completed before you tire and must stop.

Record the number in the Fitness Test Result Worksheet on page 27 and compare your number with the following chart.

Squats Fitness Determined by Age

		18-25	26–35	36–45	46–55	56–65	65+
Excellent		49+	45+	41+	35+	31+	28+
Good	No. of Squats	40–48	36–44	31–40	26–34	22–30	20–27
Average		35-39	31–35	27–30	22–25	17–21	15–19
Fair		29–34	27–30	21–26	16–21	12–16	10–14
Poor		28-	26-	20-	15-	11-	9-

FLEXIBILITY

The most commonly overlooked aspect of physical fitness is flexibility. Flexibility is the range of motion of the body's joints. Flexibility is the result of muscles, tendons and ligaments working together. People will often focus on increasing their body's muscles without taking flexibility into consideration. As muscle strength increases, the body exerts more force on the tendons and ligaments. It's important, therefore, to increase your flexibility so as to avoid injury to tendons and ligaments. You can become more flexible by stretching. Stretching should be approached with the same care and precision that you would bring to any other aspect of an exercise routine. Incorporate stretching into every workout. With increased flexibility you will be more able to increase your strength and endurance while decreasing the chance of injury. Without proper stretching, these crucial tissues can be damaged under the new strain. Stretching enables the tendons and ligaments to handle the stress and grow with the muscles.

Sit and Reach Test: The sit and reach test measures the flexibility of your hamstrings and lower back. Before you begin, make sure you warm up. Place a ruler or tape measure on the floor with the numbers increasing away from you. Sit on the floor with your legs straight so that your heels line up with the 23-inch mark. The numbers should get higher past your heels. While seated, place your hands on top of each other and stretch forward toward your toes without bouncing. Slowly reach three times and on the fourth reach record your measurement. Have someone stand over you as you reach so they can read the stretch correctly for you. The numbers listed in the table below offer median measurements. Age and arm length contribute to scoring differences.

Record results in the Fitness Test Results Worksheet on page 27 and compare your number with the following chart.

Sit and Reach Flexibility

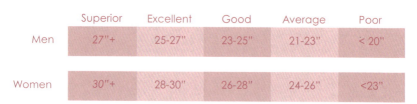

	Superior	Excellent	Good	Average	Poor
Men	27"+	25-27"	23-25"	21-23"	< 20"
Women	30"+	28-30"	26-28"	24-26"	<23"

OVERALL FITNESS RESULTS WORKSHEET

Use the following Fitness Test Results Worksheet to record the results of the tests taken in this chapter. These numbers will be used in later chapters to prepare a fitness routine with realistic and achievable goals.

Fitness Test Results Worksheet

Date: _____

TEST	INITIAL	3 MONTHS	6 MONTHS	9 MONTHS	12 MONTHS
Heart Rate (resting)					
Blood Pressure					
Body Fat %					
Body Mass Index					
Push-up					
Sit-up					
Squat					
Sit & Reach					

GETTING

AND STAYING FIT!

There are four keys to success when creating and maintaining a workout program: (1) Setting Realistic Goals, (2) Creating a Plan, (3) Keeping Track of Progress, and (4) Celebrating Achievement. Together, they will help change your lifestyle and alter your views about working out.

While each person has a different motivation for getting fit, the reasons an exercise routine fails are usually the same: burnout, injury, or failure to meet goals. Focusing on the positive aspects of working out is crucial to overcoming the mental obstacles that are common among people in any fitness program. Concentrating on the benefits you will gain from your routine is important. If you can see the evidence of your achievements, you are more likely to maintain your efforts to attain your personal fitness goals.

The way you perceive working out can impact the success of your program. Try to maintain a positive attitude during your workout program. It is important to avoid the negativity that can result if you deviate from your plan. It is very common for people just starting out to become frustrated if they don't see immediate progress or if they have to miss a session. It is important to combat negative thoughts such as "My day is ruined" by remembering that an occasional missed session is insignificant in the context of a long-term fitness routine. A missed session can be an excellent motivational tool. Refocus your energy and determination during your next workout session.

Recognize that change takes time. The keys to maintaining a fitness routine are patience, consistency and discipline. Fitness should be an ongoing endeavor. During this journey, make sure you don't lose sight of the benefits of exercise. Enjoy the changes in your body, your better mood, and increased energy. Feel the sense of accomplishment when you take positive actions towards a healthier lifestyle. Fitness is not just a goal to be reached, but rather a new way to live.

SETTING REALISTIC GOALS

Many fitness routines fail or are abandoned because of unrealistic goals. Setting unrealistic goals can make it extremely difficult to keep up with a fitness routine. It is important to consider how you phrase your fitness and exercise goals. Statements like "I'm going to lose twenty pounds in three months" are unrealistic and will most likely result in failure. It is critical to replace the results-based statements (like the one above) with statements about the effort you plan to put forth toward realistic steps to achieve fitness goals (e.g., "I will work out three times a week for at least a half an hour."). Individuals who set unrealistic goals might overexert themselves, resulting in burnout or injury. Or an individual will become discouraged after failing to meet an unrealistic expectation and give up on the routine. The bottom line is to establish a workout routine with achievable short-term and long-term goals.

By taking a realistic look at all of the factors that influence your physical fitness, you can begin to set realistic short- and long-term goals. Goals should be based on your body type, current physical condition, and life circumstances. General long-term goals can include weight loss, better endurance, or a more muscular physical appearance. Try to narrow down these broad goals so they are specific and measurable. If weight loss is a goal, determine your target weight or chose an article of clothing that you want to fit into. If you are looking to improve your endurance, make your goal completing a half marathon. After you have determined your long-term goals, break them down into more immediate ones. Use these short-term goals to track your progress and measure the success of your program. Once a short-term goal is achieved, replace it with a new one. If progress towards a goal is slow, try changing your routine to see better results. Make sure your long-term and short-term goals are attainable, yet challenging. Goals can be both physical achievements, such as hiking to the top of a local mountain, or related to the fitness routine itself—for example, completing a workout session three times a week for four straight weeks.

CREATING A PLAN

Fitness plans that work best incorporate your likes and dislikes. It is important to choose a program that is appropriate for your lifestyle and ability. If you don't feel comfortable in a gym and prefer to work out alone, chose a routine that can be accomplished at home or at a local park. You're more likely to stick with a fitness routine molded to match your lifestyle.

While every plan should be created to meet the needs of the individual, all plans should include diversity and fun. A fitness plan should contain a variety of activities. This will help prevent boredom and injury. By varying the routine, the body is forced to adapt in new ways, making an injury from an unaccustomed move or exercise less likely.

All fitness plans should include a minimum of each of the three main types of fitness programs (strength, cardiovascular and flexibility). The body cannot achieve its maximum potential unless you attend to all three types of fitness programs together. Neglecting or eliminating one of these elements can result in fatigue, decreased performance, and injury.

KEEPING TRACK OF YOUR PROGRESS

It is important to keep track of your progress. Monitoring your progress on a regular basis with the workout journal in this book will help you stay motivated, focused and disciplined. It will also help you determine the effectiveness of your routine and measure your success. Everyone's body is different; therefore, progress will vary from one person to another.

Sometimes, it may even seem like you're losing ground, but that may not be cause for concern. For example, people will often gain weight initially when beginning a fitness routine. This happens due to the increase in muscle mass. This weight gain should not be interpreted as failure, but as an indicator that your body is changing. These types of changes are why continuous monitoring is critical.

If weight loss is the main goal of a fitness program, it is logical that weight is an important measure of progress. Weight measurements should be done in the most uniform way possible. Each weighing should happen at roughly the same time of the day. For the most consistent and accurate results, weigh yourself in the morning before getting dressed.

As mentioned earlier, it is also important to set and keep track of the immediate goals regarding the frequency, intensity, and duration of your workouts. For example, if you want to gain strength, you will need to weight train two to three times a week. In this case, it is important to record how often you work out, as well as the weight, repetitions and sets for each exercise. Use the daily workout journal included in this book to keep track of your fitness routine and to make notes regarding your progress. Keeping track of your fitness routine on a daily basis will help you recognize your achievements, stay motivated, and indicate when you need to modify your program.

CELEBRATING ACHIEVEMENTS

Years of research show that reinforcement is key to incorporating new behaviors (e.g., regularly going to the gym) your life. Celebrating your achievements will increase the likelihood that you will continue with your fitness routine. Therefore, it is important to reward yourself when you make progress towards your short- and long-term goals.

Be sure to incorporate an incentive program into your fitness plan. Reward yourself only when you achieve a specific goal. For example, you might decide that going to the gym three times per week for one month deserves a reward. Achieving a certain level of weight loss might be another good milestone for earning a treat.

The type of reward you give yourself is just as important as the achievement you are celebrating. Rewards should be carefully selected to support your workout program. Rewards should be healthy and should not be something that you will obtain regardless of your results. For example, a vacation that you have already planned and paid for is not a good reward since you are going to get that whether or not you stick to your workout schedule. Instead, choose something that is extra, such as going to a movie, buying a new pair of shoes, or splurging on an expensive dinner.

HELPFUL HINTS TO GETTING AND STAYING FIT

Here are some helpful tips to starting and maintaining a fitness plan:

Schedule and plan your workouts in advance. Write down your program on a calendar a week ahead of time. Avoid saying things like "If I have time, I'll go for a run." If you plan ahead, you can fit workouts into a busy schedule.

Keep a positive attitude. Don't worry if you slip up on occasion and miss a session. Just use it as motivation to make the most of your next workout. Start the day with exercise. Those who work out in the morning enjoy the effects all day long.

Find a "fitness buddy." Your partner should be someone who has similar fitness goals. Encouragement from friends can be very motivating.

ADJUSTING ATTITUDES TOWARD FITNESS

Your attitude toward exercise is just as important as the exercise itself. The goal is to change the way you view exercise. Use the following techniques to change your mental outlook and increase the benefits of exercise.

Focus: When exercising, it is important to focus on the task at hand. Concentrating on your exercise will help you maximize the results you achieve during a session. Distraction often leads to boredom, which is one of the reasons people stop working out.

Visualization: Before beginning any fitness routine, it is helpful to attach some visual image to the routine. It is important to imagine the most specific images and sounds possible. For example, you might imagine the sound of lifting weights off the rack, and connect that image to arriving at the top of a mountain. Think about how a mountain's rocky terrain feels under your feet and how the spectacular view from the top makes you feel.

Realization: A successful workout routine is the result of willpower, determination, and the desire to accomplish your goals. As you make progress, you realize that you can achieve great things. Use this realization when you're fatigued, depressed, or bored. Knowing you have achieved something and realizing that you can do it even better the next time will lift your aspirations to new levels. Positive thinking will encourage you to persevere through moments of self-doubt and negativity.

Redirection: If you begin to doubt your abilities, simply redirect that negativity into something positive and believe in it. Replace every negative thought with a more powerful positive thought. For example, "I can't." becomes "I've succeeded already. I can do it again!"

Record changes in your mental outlook along with your physical accomplishments in the journal provided. Your newfound confidence and positive mental outlook will probably transfer to other aspects of your life. People who regularly exercise often become more patient, resistant to discouragement, and enjoy a more positive outlook on life.

PART 2: COMPONENTS OF A COMPLETE WORKOUT PROGRAM

Every fitness program should contain (1) cardiovascular, (2) strength and (3) flexibility training. While each person's body and fitness goals are different, it is important to include all three components in order to maximize the body's potential, minimize risk of injury, and avoid burnout. Training in each area enhances training in the others, resulting in optimum body performance.

CARDIOVASCULAR TRAINING

Cardiovascular training focuses on improving your heart's ability to provide oxygen to your body. By requiring muscles to perform repetitious acts with only brief moments of rest, you force your heart to adapt in order to increase the amount of oxygenated blood it pumps to the muscles. This is what is known as aerobic exercise. Aerobic exercises are performed at less-than-maximum intensity in a repetitive manner for a prolonged period of time. These activities, such as running, walking, swimming and bicycling, require oxygenated blood to be constantly delivered to the muscles. Through cardiovascular training, endurance increases and your body begins to maintain a higher and more efficient consumption of oxygen.

BENEFITS OF CARDIOVASCULAR TRAINING

Improved cardiovascular fitness means that your heart is more effective at pumping oxygenated blood throughout the body. Because the heart itself depends on a steady supply of oxygenated blood, improved blood circulation increases the heart's ability to function. Better circulation also reduces strain on the heart and lowers the risk of heart disease. Studies have also shown that improved cardiovascular fitness helps lower cholesterol levels, which decreases the chances of having a heart attack or a stroke.

Scientists are finding that those who undergo regular cardiovascular training experience physical benefits beyond those related to the heart and other muscles. Increased blood flow to major organs helps promote a healthy body. Regular aerobic exercise can help maintain your body's bone mass. Recent studies have shown that dieting to lose fat rapidly may also result in a significant loss in bone density unless you exercise regularly. Those who maintain a regular cardiovascular training routine can even increase bone density. By increasing bone density, you decrease your risk of developing a serious weakening of bones, known as osteoporosis.

Those who maintain a fitness routine that includes cardiovascular training enjoy both physical and mental benefits. The increase in activity results in weight loss, enhanced muscular endurance, improved blood circulation, and superior heart and lung capacity. The process also stimulates the production of endorphins, naturally occurring substances that are associated with elevated mood and stress reduction.

DIFFERENT TYPES OF CARDIOVASCULAR TRAINING

Cardiovascular training varies in its degree of impact, level of intensity, and duration of exercise. These factors should be weighed before you select a fitness routine. The current condition of your body will help determine the proper type of cardio training for you.

Impact is the degree to which your body experiences the force of gravity. Activities that are considered high impact, like running, require your body to absorb the force of its weight as your feet hit the ground. High impact activities are excellent cardio exercises and can be done anywhere. However, people who have poor joints or who are recovering from injury should avoid high impact exercise. A strained back or sore knee will be made worse by the constant impact of the body's weight hitting the ground.

Those suffering from injuries should consider some form of low impact cardio workout. Low impact exercises involve little or no jarring. Swimming is an excellent low impact cardiovascular activity that utilizes all major muscles groups. Bicycling is also considered a low impact activity, although it emphasizes building up the lower body.

Intensity refers to the amount of energy that is used during an exercise and determines your heart rate and blood pressure. The higher the level of intensity, the more your heart will be forced to work. While higher intensity activities (e.g., running) have greater results than low intensity work-outs (walking) over the same time-period, they may pose serious health risks to people who suffer from high blood pressure or who have been sedentary for a long time. Exercises should be performed at a level of intensity that is challenging but within your capabilities. The intensity of an exercise should be at a level that can be maintained throughout the duration of the routine.

Duration is the amount of time you exercise for any given period. Most experts agree that an individual should exercise for at least thirty minutes' duration three times a week. Individuals just starting a cardio routine should begin by following this guideline. Select activities that you can sustain throughout the exercise period.

HOW TO DETERMINE YOUR CARDIOVASCULAR PERFORMANCE

In order to improve your cardiovascular system's performance, you must first determine your target heart rate. Your target heart rate is the range where your body is able to most efficiently increase cardiovascular fitness.

The first step in finding your target heart rate, then, is to determine your maximum heart rate. Your maximum heart rate is a function of your age. In order to determine your maximum heart rate, enter your age into the equation below:

220 – Age = Maximum Heart Rate

For example, if you are forty-four years of age, your maximum heart rate will be 176.

The following chart shows the range of target and maximum heart rates by age.

Target and Maximum Heart Rates Determined by Age

AGE	TARGET HEART RATE (50-85% OF MHR)	MAXIMUM HEART RATE
20	100-170	200
25	98-166	195
30	95-162	190
35	93-157	185
40	90-153	180
45	88-149	175
50	85-145	170
55	83-140	165
60	80-136	160
65	78-132	155
70	75-128	150

There are three heart rate zones that focus on specific aspects of cardiovascular performance. These three zones are endurance, aerobic, and anaerobic. By targeting any one of these zones, you can control the benefits you get from cardiovascular exercise. The following table illustrates the range of these zones and their benefits.

Heart Rate Zones

ZONE	% OF MAXIMUM HEART RATE	PROCESS	BENEFITS
Endurance Zone	60-70%	Burning fuel with oxygen (easy)	Builds endurance & helps with fat burning
Aerobic Zone	70-80%	Burning fuel with oxygen (intense)	Improves cardiovascular system, muscles learn to utilize oxygen more efficiently
Anaerobic Zone	80-90%	Burning fuel without oxygen	Builds heart and lung capacity

CARDIOVASCULAR TRAINING FOR DIFFERENT RESULTS

By varying the duration and intensity of a workout session, you can aim to achieve specific results. For example, to lose weight effectively, you should maintain an exercise program that focuses on endurance. This means engaging in low intensity exercise over long periods of time. It takes approximately twenty minutes of aerobic exercise before the body begins to burn stored fat. If you're a beginner or are recovering from an injury, you should exercise at a low intensity for twenty minutes, three times a week. In this case it may take some time before you lose any fat. As your body becomes stronger, you should increase the duration and intensity of your workouts.

If you are one of those individuals who are looking to gain weight, you should not skip cardiovascular training. Instead, you should include a routine that does not hinder you from achieving your fitness goals. Two, twenty-minute, low intensity sessions will help strengthen the heart without causing weight loss.

Many people, of course, choose overall cardiovascular fitness as their goal. Exercise for between twenty and forty minutes at least three times a week in the aerobic zone if you want to increase your overall cardiovascular performance.

Both high intensity training and low intensity training burn fat. Low intensity activities, those where the heart rate is between 60 and 70 percent of the maximum, burn fat at a low, steady level. However, high intensity activities, where the heart rate is between 70 and 85 percent of the maximum, burn calories faster, allowing you to make the most of your workout. Higher intensity activities also have a lasting effect on your metabolism, resulting in an increase in calories burned even when you're not exercising.

GUIDELINES FOR SUCCESSFUL CARDIOVASCULAR TRAINING

In order to maximize the benefits of cardiovascular training, you should consider not only when and where to work out, but also how long you'll exercise and in what order you'll do your exercises. The following guidelines will help you prepare your cardio workout routine.

Workout schedule: Many people find that working out in the morning gives them a boost in energy that lasts throughout the day. Others find exercising in the early evening helps prepare them for sleep. When you work out is up to you. Select a routine that best fits your lifestyle.

Warm-up and cool-down: All workouts should be preceded by a warm-up and followed by a cool-down. Warm-ups prepare your body for the stress it's about to undergo. Cool-downs gradually bring you back to a resting state and release muscle tension that could lead to soreness.

Footwear: Improper footwear can result in discomfort, blisters and serious injury. Most specialty footwear stores will measure your feet carefully in order to find a shoe that fits exactly. Your shoes should feel good as soon as you try them on; do not buy uncomfortable shoes with the expectation that they'll get more comfortable after they're broken in. Exercise footwear should be used for exercise only. You should replace your shoes according to the schedule suggested by the manufacturer.

Double Session: Individuals will often combine strength and cardiovascular training in one workout session. Start out with strength training and follow that with cardiovascular exercise to get the best results from both. If cardiovascular training is done first, muscle fatigue severely diminishes your ability to lift at your full capacity. By strength training first, you increase the efficiency of your cardiovascular workout because your heart rate will have already entered the fat-burning zone. You'll have saved yourself the 20 minutes of continuous cardio exercise necessary for your body to start burning fat for energy.

Pace: Speed and intensity should be maintained at a level that does not hurt. Use your own comfort level to determine when you should increase the intensity and speed of your exercise. The pace should be challenging, slightly uncomfortable, but never painful.

Variation: In order to maximize results and prevent uneven muscular development, exercise routines should be varied so as to involve all the different parts of the body.

Frequency: A successful cardiovascular fitness routine consists of working out 3-4 days a week for 20 to 60 minutes.

CALORIES BURNED FOR CARDIOVASCULAR ACTIVITY

The rate at which calories are burned is determined by the intensity of the activity. Refer to the tables listed on pages 62-63, which show the number of calories burned per hour by average adults for various aerobic activities.

SAMPLE CARDIOVASCULAR PROGRAM

Experts recommend that people should engage in at least twenty to thirty minutes of cardiovascular training three or four times a week. Below are two calendars showing examples of high and low intensity workout regimens. These exercise programs should only be used as guides in creating a personalized fitness plan. An ideal fitness plan should become a part of your life. Therefore, it is important that you choose activities for your routine that you will enjoy. This will help you maintain your momentum and enthusiasm for the whole program.

Sample Low Intensity Workouts

LOW INTENSITY WORKOUTS						
Sunday	Monday	Tuesday	Wednesday	Thursday	Friday	Saturday
		20 min walk during lunch break		30 min stationary bike		2 mile hike
	20 min walk before work				30 min swimming	
25 min walk to store for newspaper		take stairs instead of elevator	30 min walk during son's soccer practice			1 round of golf with hand cart
	30 min aerobics			40 min yoga	25 min walk before work	
		30 min swimming		30 min walk at the mall		

Sample Low and High Intensity Workouts

HIGH INTENSITY WORKOUTS						
Sunday	Monday	Tuesday	Wednesday	Thursday	Friday	Saturday
	30 min run (street)		25 min spinning (stationary bike)		vigorous mountain hike	
30 min swimming		25 min stationary step climber				1 round of golf with hand cart
	30 min basketball with co-workers			30 min run before work		60 min dancing at wedding reception
40 min bicycle ride		20 min climb stairs during lunch break		35 min stationary elliptical trainer		
40 min rollerblading			25 min spinning (stationary bike)			

CARDIOVASCULAR ASSESSMENT WORKSHEET

In order to track your success you must determine your baseline cardiovascular fitness. This information will help you decide the level of exercise that is right for you. In order to complete the worksheet you will have to perform a minimum of twenty minutes of either low or high impact aerobic exercise. You can find a chart on page 39 that will help you calculate your Maximum Heart Rate and Target Heart Rate. You can find your Heart Rate Zone in the table on page 40.

Resting Heart Rate _____

Maximum Heart Rate _____

Target Heart Rate _____

Selected Activity _____

Duration _____

Active Heart Rate _____

Heart Rate Zone _____

STRENGTH TRAINING

Strength training involves overloading your muscles in order to increase their strength and ability to do work. Strength training is an anaerobic activity, meaning that during this type of exercise your muscles don't consume oxygen. These are explosive activities (jump squats, weight lifting, etc.,) that focus on increasing intensity and strength. Strength training involves keeping the targeted muscles activated near or at their maximum capacity for a short period.

BENEFITS OF STRENGTH TRAINING

There are many reasons why you should incorporate strength training into your workout program. Strength training increases the durability of bones, muscles, tendons and ligaments, making your body less susceptible to injury. It can also increase bone density and may help prevent osteoporosis. Recent studies have uncovered convincing evidence that strength training reduces cholesterol, resulting in a lower risk of heart disease. With a regular strength training routine, you will see increases in lean muscle mass and metabolism. In addition, stronger muscles help improve balance, mobility and endurance. Your figure or posture will also improve as your skeletal muscles help you stand up straighter. Strength training also helps bolster mental health by reducing stress and improving self-esteem. Resistance training has also been proven to increase the body's production of chemicals known as neurotransmitters (dopamine, serotonin and norepinephrine), which act on the pleasure centers of the brain, increasing feelings of contentment and well-being.

DIFFERENT TYPES OF STRENGTH TRAINING

Strength training involves exerting force by pushing, pulling or lifting objects of varying weight. Two other factors that strength training takes into account are the frequency and duration of the exercise. The three most common forms of strength training are:

Weight Training: Through the lifting and lowering of weights, muscles are overloaded. This forces them to grow. Each weight training exercise consists of three alterable components:

Weight: The level of force acting against the muscle.

Repetitions: The number of times the weight is lifted and lowered without resting.

Sets: Series of repetitions grouped together. Specific routines differ according to the number of sets they include.

Utilize different numbers of sets, repetitions and weight during your workout to make progress toward specific goals. Generally, high resistance with a small number of repetitions is used to increase muscle size and strength. More repetitions using a lower weight increases muscular endurance, tone, and definition without adding bulk.

Resistance Training: This is the use of elastic or hydraulic (water) resistance to force required muscles to work. Resistance training applies the same principles as weight training, but uses elastic exercise bands or water (usually in a swimming pool) instead of gravity to stress the muscles. Resistance training differs from weight training with regard to when the muscles experience the greatest stress. In training with hand weights or free weights, the largest amount of force is applied to the muscle at the start of each repetition. Elastic resistance causes the greatest amount of resistance at the end of the rep, when the elastic is stretched to its limit. Hydraulic resistance works against the muscle uniformly during the entire repetition. Most gyms have some resistance training machines, but if you buy elastic bands you can do resistance training almost anywhere.

Isometric Training: This type of exercise engages the muscle in a fixed position. Isometric training or isometrics, such as holding yourself in a push-up position, fully activates the muscles while your joints and overall position remain stable. Be careful with this type of training, since the large amount of weight and the static nature of the exercise make it possible to seriously injure yourself. Professional instruction is recommended before undertaking strenuous isometric exercises.

Form is the most overlooked and arguably the most important aspect of strength training. Since strength training relies on the isolation and overloading of specific muscles, it is essential to learn proper form. People who do not learn proper form will see little increase in strength. They also risk serious injuries. Make an appointment with a personal trainer if you are unfamiliar with strength training. A professional accredited trainer can help you perfect your form and guide you through a personalized strength-training program.

CORRECT ORDER FOR TRAINING MAJOR MUSCLE GROUPS

It is important to exercise muscles in the correct order to maximize the benefits of each exercise. The correct order involves working from groups of larger muscles to smaller muscles. If smaller muscles are worked first they become fatigued. As a result, the large muscles will not be able to work at their optimum level.

Abdominals: Targeting the abdominals first is important in order to prevent injury. Strong abdominal muscles will help stabilize your body so all other muscle groups can be exercised properly.

Lower Body (quadriceps, gluteus maximus, hamstring, calf, etc): These are large muscles that will help promote blood flow through your body, essentially warming the rest of your body up and preparing it for working out.

Chest: When working the chest muscles, focus on engaging the pectoral muscles rather than relying on those in your arms. Improper form can overwork the biceps, triceps and shoulder muscles.

Back (upper and lower): Work both the upper and lower back. Focus on using the muscles of the back while stabilizing your body with your abdominal muscles and guiding the weight with your arms.

Shoulder: Shoulders (deltoids) are often the most overlooked and incorrectly exercised area of the body. Increase weight slowly and use exercises that isolate the different areas of the shoulders such as the front (anterior), middle (medial) and back (posterior).

Arms (Triceps and Biceps): Working the arms too early in your routine will decrease the muscles' ability to perform. Be sure your routine is arranged so you have enough energy to complete your entire workout. It is better to do fewer sets and complete the entire circuit than to neglect a muscle group.

Figure: Outline of Body Front/Back Showing Main Muscle Groups

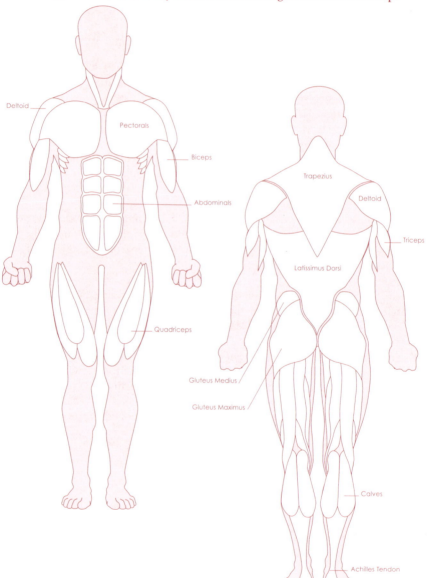

STRENGTH TRAINING FOR INDIVIDUAL NEEDS

Modify your strength training routine to suit your individual goals.

In order to increase muscle mass and build up large muscles, use heavy weights with a low number of repetitions. The weight should be heavy enough so that it is difficult to lift, but leaves you able to complete your last rep. Rest periods should increase, allowing the muscles to work at or close to their maximum capability.

To increase tone and muscle definition, weight should be decreased and the number of repetitions increased.

To increase muscular endurance, weight should be lowered further and repetitions and sets increased. Rest time should also be decreased, forcing the muscle to engage more frequently with less rest.

The following charts are examples of weight, repetitions, sets and other information for specific muscle development.

Information on Strength Training for Desired Effects

	BUILD LARGER MUSCLE	TONE & DEFINE	MUSCULAR ENDURANCE
% of maximum weight	80-100	60-80	40-60
Repetitions per set	1-5	8-15	25-60
Sets per exercise	3-5	4-8	2-4
Rest between sets (mins)	2-6	2-5	1-2
Duration (seconds per set)	4-8	20-60	80-150
Speed per rep (% of max)	90-100	60-90	60-80
Training sessions per week	3-6	5-7	8-14

All workout routines should be approached cautiously. Everyone reacts differently to strength training and therefore you should proceed at your own pace. It is better to start slow and work out longer, rather than overexert yourself and quit early. Gradually incorporate strength training into your routine. Focus on correct form and allow enough time for muscles to recover. Proper form helps you see faster results and diminishes your risk of injury. Concentrate on using strength instead of momentum to lift a weight and lower it. If you have never weight trained, it's a good idea to work with a personal trainer to learn the correct technique for each exercise.

It is important to prepare your body for weight training. Engage in ten minutes of light aerobic activity and stretching to warm up. Exerting yourself too soon may result in decreased performance and injury. Begin with one exercise per muscle group. Gradually increase the reps, the number of exercises and the weight for each session until you reach your desired goal.

STRENGTH TRAINING ACTIVITY CHART

Weight training should be done between 2 and 3 times a week. Allow at least a day's rest after a day in which you exercise. Begin by performing

Typical Beginners Strength Training Routine

ACTIVITY	MUSCLE GROUP	SETS	REPS
Crunch Machine	Abdominals (front)	1	15-30
Dumbel Side Bend	Abdominals (side)	1 (each side)	15-30
Squats	Lower Body	4	8-12
Bench Press	Chest	4	8-12
Lat Pull Down	Back	4	8-12
Shoulder Press	Shoulders	4	8-12
Curl	Biceps	4	8-12
Rope Pulley Triceps Extension	Triceps	4	8-12

1 or 2 sets per exercise, depending on the weight. Make sure you get the maximum results from each exercise by using proper form and technique. The table on the previous page is an example of a typical beginner's weight training regimen. Select a weight that is challenging, but manageable.

STRENGTH ASSESSMENT WORKSHEET

In order to track your individual progress, it is important to ascertain your baseline strength. This information will be useful when you decide on your first daily goals in the Daily Workout Journal. To find your baseline strength, select a weight that you can lift at least ten or more times and continue lifting it until you must stop from fatigue. Whenever you are lifting weights, it is important to keep safety in mind. It is best to exercise with a partner who can "spot" the weight and help keep you safe. Record your results on the worksheet that follows.

Baseline Strength Assessment Worksheet

Activity	Weight	Repetitions
Abdominal Crunch Machine	_____	_____
Squat Press	_____	_____
Bench Press	_____	_____
Lat Pull Down	_____	_____
Bicep Curl	_____	_____
Triceps Press	_____	_____

NOTES

FLEXIBILITY TRAINING

Flexibility training, or stretching, manipulates your joints, muscles, tendons and ligaments in order to increase their range of motion. Increasing your flexibility strengthens these elements of your anatomy, improves your overall performance and helps prevent injury. Flexibility training may consist of slow, fluid motions that target specific locations on a joint's range of motion, or it may involve rapid, sweeping movements that target the entire range of motion.

BENEFITS OF FLEXIBILITY TRAINING

Regular flexibility training or stretching helps increase circulation, prevent injury, decrease stress and improve joint movement. Stretching increases muscular elasticity, which allows muscles to function better under stress and achieve higher levels of performance. Increased flexibility aligns your body by strengthening the tendons, ligaments, and muscles that maintain your shape and posture. Stronger tendons and ligaments help prevent muscles from becoming strained or knotted. Proper stretching reduces muscle tension and helps alleviate stress.

DIFFERENT TYPES OF FLEXIBILITY TRAINING

Flexibility training focuses on your joints in order to increase their strength and range of motion. This is accomplished through manipulating the force exerted against the joint and the duration of the stretch. The most common forms of flexibility training are:

Passive stretching: With this type of flexibility training, an external force stretches the joint to its most extreme position while the body's muscles remain loose. The split is an example of passive stretching. The stretch is kept at full extension for 10 to 30 seconds before being gently released. Passive stretching can be accomplished with the help of a partner or an inanimate object, such as a chair, floor, or wall.

Static stretching: This type of flexibility training utilizes opposing muscle groups to hold the stretch in place. The most common example of static stretching is touching one's toes. Static stretching involves moving slowly toward the extreme position of a joint and holding that position for 10 to 30 seconds. As your body relaxes the joint will become more flexible, allowing for an increase in the joint's range of motion.

Isometric stretching: With this type of flexibility training, an external force immobilizes the joint at its full extension while the muscles are alternately contracted and relaxed. A good example of an isometric stretch is the "wall-calf stretch," in which you place your hands against a wall and actively push against it while engaging your calf muscle. Assume a passive stretch position and then tense the muscle between five and fifteen seconds. Then release it and allow it to relax for at least twenty seconds. No movement should occur during isometric stretching. Due to the strain placed on the body's ligaments, isometric stretching should be done only after you are thoroughly warmed up. Young children and the elderly should avoid isometric stretching.

Dynamic stretching: This type of flexibility training exploits the joint's full range of motion. This form of stretching uses speed and momentum to achieve the stretch. Unlike other forms of stretching, dynamic stretching does not hold the stretch, but rather focuses on the fluid movements of your body. Examples of dynamic stretching include trunk twists and high kicks. These stretches are often used for improving flexibility for specific joints and can be tailored to mimic specific tasks required for particular sports (e.g., a tennis player may perform a mock serve without a racket or ball).

DETERMINING YOUR BODY'S FLEXIBILITY

Your flexibility is determined by your overall condition and genetic predispositions. However, you can improve your flexibility within these limits by stretching on a daily basis. Every person has a different potential for flexibility, but we all share common internal and external factors that increase or limit our flexibility:

Elasticity: The elasticity of connective tissues like muscles, fascia, tendons and ligaments provides the most direct opportunity for improving flexibility. Through proper training, connective tissue can attain greater elasticity, which results in improved flexibility.

Muscle function: A muscle's ability to correctly and efficiently contract is essential to your flexibility. Strength training helps build stronger muscles and therefore promotes flexibility.

External factors: Flexibility can be impeded by injury to the muscles and other connective tissues. Flexibility can also vary by age, degree of physical activity, the amount of water and minerals (such as potassium) within the body, and the amount of fatty tissue in the body.

Average Range of Motion of Typical Adults

JOINT	ROTATION	RANGE OF MOTION (IN DEGREES)
Neck	Head rotation (look toward the left & right)	70-90 both directions
Neck	Head tilt forward (look down)	30-85
Neck	Head tilt backward (look up)	30-75
Neck	Side head tilt (look front, tilt head right & left)	30-45 both directions
Back	Rotate trunk to right & left	5-30
Back	Tilt trunk from one side to the other from waist	15-25 both directions
Back	Tilt froward from waist towards toes	45-60
Back	Lean backwards from waist	25
Shoulder	Arms straight, downward, make tight circles	0-180
Shoulder	Arms straight, out to side, make tight circles	0-180
Elbow	Fully extended then bend to fully flexed	0/135 degrees
Forearm	Rotation (keep wrist immobile)	180
Wrist	Hands palms down, extend fingertips to sky	70
Wrist	Hands palms down, extend fingertips to ground	80
Wrist	Hands palms down tilt thumb toward forearms	20
Wrist	Hands palms down, tilt pinky toward forearms	45
Hip	On back, lift legs, point toes up, rotate a straight leg toward head	125 both legs
Hip	On stomach with toes pointed toward the ground, lift heel to point up	0-30 both legs
Hip	Sit legs together, toes pointed up, rotate one leg out while leg remains straight, toes point up	0-45 both legs
Knee	Straighten leg, bend knee, bring heel to thigh	140
Ankle	Foot perpendicular to leg, bring toes toward shin	20
Ankle	Foot perpendicular to leg, extend toes from body	50

GUIDELINES FOR SUCCESSFUL FLEXIBILITY TRAINING

In order to implement a successful flexibility training routine, consider the following guidelines:

Breathing: Focus on your breathing. Start with an inhalation, and then slowly exhale while you stretch.

Warm-up and cool-down: Flexibility training during warm-up and cool-down periods should be part of every strength and cardiovascular training session. A warm-up allows the body to prepare for the stress of exercise, while a cool-down allows the body to release stress and return to its resting state.

Avoid overstretching: Overstretching can weaken, injure, or damage the body just as much as overexertion can. Pay attention to your body's signals and stop all exercise if stretching becomes painful.

Bouncing or ballistic stretching: Avoid sudden jerking or bouncing during stretching. Sudden, jarring movements can increase the chance of injury. All stretching motion should be fluid, without abrupt starts and stops.

Comfort level: Stretches should be take you beyond your normal comfort levels, but not to the point of pain. You should experience only mild discomfort while stretching.

Holding: Every stretch should be held for at least 8 seconds, unless the stretch is dynamic.

SAMPLE FLEXIBILITY PROGRAM

A proper flexibility training program targets all major muscle groups and their corresponding joints. The routine provided in the following table is an example of a typical warm-up stretch.

Typical Warm-up Stretches

STRETCH	DESCRIPTION
Shoulder Shrugs	Raise shoulders towards ears. Hold for 5 seconds before releasing. Tension should be felt in the neck and shoulders.
Chest Stretch	Take hold of stationary object with both hands. Keep feet planted. Turn left or right, open chest. Stretch should be felt in chest, shoulder and bicep. Hold 10 seconds. Repeat in other direction.
Arm/ Shoulder	Place right hand on left arm just below the elbow. Move left arm against body and while right arm pulls inward, push left arm against right hand. Hold for 10 seconds and repeat on opposite side.
Triceps	Grab left elbow with right hand. Pull elbow inward and bend at the hips toward the right. Hold for 10 seconds and repeat on opposite side.
Abdominal	Lie on stomach. Push up with arms. Keep hips firm to the floor while head lifts towards sky. Hold for 15 seconds and repeat.
Calf	In front of a wall stand with one foot 2-3 feet in front of the other. Bend the front leg until the back leg becomes straight. Move hips forward until encountering tension. Hold 10-15 seconds, release, repeat with oppostie foot forward.
Spine	Sit on ground with legs forward. Bring right foot over left leg slightly above knee. Place right hand flat on ground behind. Twisting from the waist, rotate the spine and body to the right. Allow the neck to rotate the head so eyes look behind. Hold for 15 seconds, release and repeat on the other side.
Thigh	Stand on one leg with other leg folded back so heel touches the buttocks. Using your hand take the ankle of the folded leg, pull up. Hold for 10 seconds. Release and repeat on opposite leg.
Hamstring	From the standing position, bend at the hips extending the arms down and allow the fingers to touch the toes.

FLEXIBILITY ASSESSMENT WORKSHEET

In order to track your individual progress, it is important to determine your baseline flexibility. You can use this information as you set daily goals in the Daily Workout Journal beginning on page 125. Select an intensity that will allow you to hold a stretch for at least five to eight seconds. Eventually, you should be able to hold a stretch between five and fifteen seconds. Record the length of time for each stretch. Also note your level of discomfort from one to ten, with one being no pain and ten being pain so intense that it causes you to abandon the stretch.

Fitness Test Results Worksheet

Date: _____

ACTIVITY	REACH	HOLD TIME	LEVEL OF DISCOMFORT
Shoulder Shrug			
Chest Stretch			
Arm/Shoulder			
Triceps/Back			
Abdominal			
Calf			
Thigh			
Hamstring			

CALORIES AND
PHYSICAL ACTIVITIES

We burn the calories that food provides in the course of exercising and in our daily activities. Even when we're sleeping, we burn some calories. The more vigorous the activity, the more calories we burn.

Depending on what kind of work we do or what activities we engage in at home, we may use up a lot of calories during the day. The following table shows the amount of calories burned during typical daily activities. You can use this chart to calculate the approximate number of calories you burn in the course of a day. In later chapters, this book will examine how to balance the number of calories you take in against the number of calories you burn. This information will help you make healthy choices when it comes to planning a diet.

Calories Burned for Typical Physical Activities

LIGHT ACTIVITIES - 150 or less	CAL/HR
Billiards	140
Lying down/sleeping	60
Office work	140
Sitting	80
Standing	100

For most of us, our jobs and other day-to-day activities don't involve enough exercise to use up the calories we get from the food we eat. Without regular exercise, we are likely to put on weight. That weight, unfortunately, will be in the form of fat. The following table shows the number of calories you can expect to burn for each hour of moderate and vigorous activities. If you incorporate moderate or vigorous exercise into your daily routine, you can expect not only to control your weight, but to become more fit.

Calories Burned for Typical Physical Activities

MODERATE ACTIVITIES - 150-350	CAL/HR
Aerobic dancing	340
Ballroom dancing	210
Bicycling (5 mph)	170
Bowling	160
Canoeing (2.5 mph)	170
Dancing (social)	210
Gardening (moderate)	270
Golf (with cart)	180
Golf (without cart)	320
Grocery shopping	180
Horseback riding (sitting trot)	250
Light housework/cleaning, etc.	250
Ping-pong	270
Swimming (20 yards/min)	290
Tennis (recreational doubles)	310
Vacuuming	220
Volleyball (recreational)	260
Walking (2 mph)	200
Walking (3 mph)	240
Walking (4 mph)	300

Calories Burned for Typical Physical Activities

VIGOROUS ACTIVITIES - 350 or MORE	CAL/HR
Aerobics (step)	440
Backpacking (10 lb load)	540
Badminton	450
Basketball (competitive)	660
Basketball (leisure)	390
Bicycling (10 mph)	375
Bicycling (13 mph)	600
Cross country skiing (leisurely)	460
Cross country skiing (moderate)	660
Hiking	460
Ice skating (9 mph)	384
Jogging (5 mph)	550
Jogging (6 mph)	690
Racquetball	620
Rollerblading	384
Rowing machine	540
Running (8 mph)	900
Scuba diving	570
Shoveling snow	580
Soccer	580
Spinning	650
Stair climber machine	480
Swimming (50 yards/min.)	680
Water aerobics	400
Water skiing	480
Weight training (30 sec. between sets)	760
Weight training (60 sec. between sets)	570

PART 3: THINGS YOU SHOULD KNOW ABOUT NUTRITION

Proper nutrition is essential for maintaining a successful fitness routine. Food and supplemental nutrients are fuel for your body and will give you the energy to get through your workouts. Improper nutrition deprives your body of essential vitamins and minerals and limits your potential for improving your fitness. By altering your eating habits and learning how to make healthy food choices, you can see results faster and maximize the benefits of physical exercise.

NOTES

BASICS FOR EATING HEALTHY

Healthy eating is essential to improving your overall fitness. A proper, balanced diet will enable you to maximize your efforts and reach higher levels of fitness. By focusing on scientifically proven dietary guidelines, you will learn what types of foods are good for you and how much you should eat.

DIETARY GUIDELINES

Dietary guidelines published by the federal government are scientifically developed suggestions for ideal diets based on age, gender and physical activity. These guidelines show not only the types of foods and quantities people should eat, but also how they should prepare the food. These guidelines also suggest the level of activity people should strive for in order to maintain optimum health.

Start your diet planning by using the chart below to figure out your daily caloric needs. Then use the following food group charts to plan a healthy diet that meets your nutritional requirements. Your diet should include a balance of protein, carbohydrates and fats from healthful sources. You may find later that you need to modify your intake based on your fitness progress.

SUGGESTED CALORIC INTAKE

Determining how many calories you need is essential to determining what types of food and how much food to eat. The following chart estimates the ideal daily calorie consumption for individuals by age and gender.

Caloric Intake of Moderately Active Individuals

GENDER	AGE (years)	CALORIES
Female	19-30	2,000-2,200
	31-50	1,800-2,000
	51+	1,600-1,800
Male	19-30	2,600-2,800
	31-50	2,400-2,600
	51+	2,200-2,400

MAJOR FOOD GROUPS

All essential foods fall into one of six basic food groups. Essential foods provide specific nutrients that are required to maintain a healthy body. When eaten in correct proportions, these foods can improve your health, physical performance and overall well being.

Grains: These are foods that are derived from the seeds of plants such as wheat, corn, rye, oats and rice. Grains can be either whole or refined. Whole grains are an important source of nutrients such as vitamins, minerals, fiber, and protein. Whole grains include the entire grain kernel, while the refining process removes the outer coating and the germ, taking away many of the nutrients. Experts suggest that at least half of the grains we eat be whole. Check the nutrition label and look for the words "whole grain" near the top of the list. There are a lot of products that claim they are made with whole grain. However, many of these are mostly made from processed flours and only include a small amount of whole grain.

Vegetables: Choose from any vegetable in any form - cooked, raw, or even in the form of juice. Experts say you should vary the types of vegetables you eat, but suggest focusing on dark green and orange vegetables, since they have important nutrients such as folic acid and vitamin A. Experts also recommend eating dried peas and beans, since they are rich in protein and fiber.

Fruits: Fruits are an important source of vitamins and fiber. Experts recommend concentrating on fresh fruits when possible. However, frozen, canned (with as little added sugar as possible), or dried fruits can also suffice. Fruit juices should be minimized because they tend to be high in sugar. Try to vary the types of fruit you eat in order to get as many different nutrients as possible.

Milk and dairy products: Studies show that milk and dairy products are an important source of vitamin D and calcium. Milk and other dairy products can be high in saturated fats, though, so experts recommend that you focus on fat-free or low fat products. If you are lactose-intolerant, you can use supplements that help you digest lactose.

Meat: Meats are excellent sources of protein. Because meats can also contain fat, nutritionists recommend that you focus on lean meats such as fish and poultry. Avoid preparing meats by frying, since that adds unnecessary calories. Baking or grilling will help minimize the amount of fat you get with your meat.

Fats and oils: Fats in small amounts are necessary for your body to function properly. However, it's important to avoid consuming large amounts of butter and margarine because they either contain cholesterol or encourage your body to produce cholesterol. For healthier alternatives, cook with oils such as canola or olive oil. These oils contain no cholesterol.

The following table shows the amounts from each food group you should eat in order to have a balanced diet at various levels of daily caloric intake.

Daily Amount of Food From Each Food Category

CALORIES	1000	1500	2000	2500	3000
Fruits	1 cup	1.5 cups	2 cups	2 cups	2.5 cups
Vegetables	1 cup	2 cups	2.5 cups	3.5 cups	4 cups
Grains	3 oz	5 oz	6 oz	9 oz	10 oz
Meat and Beans	2 oz	5 oz	5.5 oz	6.5 oz	7 oz
Milk	2 cups	3 cups	3 cups	3 cups	3 cups
Oils	3 tsp	5 tsp	6 tsp	8 tsp	10 tsp

SERVING SIZES AND PORTION CONTROL

Healthy eating does not necessarily mean giving up the foods you like. In fact, studies show that diets that force people to stop eating their favorite foods or that keep them from enjoying an occasional restaurant meal often fail because people end up "cheating." Instead of denying yourself your favorite foods, try to limit the amounts of high-calorie foods that you consume. When you do indulge in a favorite, high-calorie snack, be sure to note the serving sizes listed on the package. Even a small package may contain several servings; avoid yielding to the temptation to consume the entire package.

When you eat at home, you can easily control the size of your portions. Restaurant meals present more of a problem. Research shows that restaurants tend to serve portions that are far larger than necessary. When eating a meal at your favorite restaurant, you can avoid overeating by simply dividing the entrée in half. You can take the other half home to eat at another meal.

ENCOURAGING BETTER FOOD CHOICES

The federal government is committed to helping people develop healthy eating habits. In 1994 Congress passed the Nutrition Labeling and Education Act (NLEA), which required that most foods, with the exception of meats and poultry, carry a nutritional facts label. These labels indicate the calories and approximate nutritional values for each serving of the food product. By learning how to read and use the nutritional label, you can make better food choices.

The nutritional label shows more than how many calories and other nutrients a food contains; it also shows the percentage of the recommended daily values of various nutrients, such as fat, carbohydrates, and protein, the food provides. The label also lists the percentage of the recommended daily values for cholesterol, sodium, and various vitamins and minerals that a serving of the food provides. These percentages are based on a 2000-calorie diet; if your diet is higher or lower in calories, the percentages will be different.

Nutrition Facts
Serving Size 1 cup (228g)
Servings Per Container 2

Amount per Serving

Calories 250   Calories from Fat 110

	% Daily Value*
Total Fat 12g	**18%**
Saturated Fat 3g	**15%**
Trans Fat 3g	
Cholesterol 30mg	**10%**
Sodium 470mg	**20%**
Total Carbohydrate 31g	**10%**
Dietary Fiber 0g	**0%**
Sugars 5g	
Protein 5g	

Vitamin A	4%
Vitamin C	2%
Calcium	20%
Iron	4%

* Percent Daily Values are based on a 2,000 calorie diet. Your Daily Values may be higher or lower depending on your calorie needs.

	Calories:	2,000	2,500
Total Fat	Less than	65g	80g
Sat Fat	Less than	20g	25g
Cholesterol	Less than	300mg	300mg
Sodium	Less than	2,400mg	2,400mg
Total Carbohydrate		300g	375g
Dietary Fiber		25g	30g

THE RELATIONSHIP BETWEEN FOOD AND FITNESS

All too often, people seeking to increase their fitness overlook the crucial role food plays in meeting their goals. Improper nutrition can deprive the body of energy, contribute to the breakdown of muscles, and undo the benefits of a fitness routine. By learning how food affects your body, you can construct a diet that helps you reach your fitness goals.

FOOD AS YOUR ENERGY SOURCE

Your body requires energy to maintain its basic functions and allow you to perform the activities that are part of your daily life. If you eat too little, you won't have the energy to get through your day—never mind working out. However, if you eat too much, your body will store the excess food as fat. The key to maintaining a healthy weight, then, is finding a balance between your activity level and the amount of food you eat.

BASEL METABOLIC RATE

Your body uses a certain amount of energy every day, even while it's at rest. This is what's known as your Basal Metabolic Rate (BMR). The Basal Metabolic Rate is the number of calories required each day to maintain normal body function. This typically represents about 70 percent of all calories consumed. Your BMR depends on a number of factors, including your gender, height, weight, and age.

Your lifestyle also has a significant effect on your BMR. People who maintain a regular fitness routine and eat properly enjoy higher BMRs since they tend to have more lean muscle and less fat than sedentary people have. Muscle tissue is "metabolically active," meaning that muscles burn calories while at rest. Conversely, those who undergo crash diets and forego exercise will have lower BMRs. This relationship between diet and exercise in determining your BMR means that you are unlikely to lose weight effectively with a crash diet. While these types of dieters may lose weight initially, they often end up gaining the weight back (and maybe even more) as their BMR drops. The key to achieving a healthy weight, then, is to stay active and pay attention to your nutrition.

FOOD QUALITY, QUANTITY AND TIMING

Proper nutrition is not only determined by what you eat, but also by how much you eat and when. The body functions best when it is provided with the proper amount of high quality food at regular intervals. Consider the following characteristics of proper nutrition when planning your diet:

Quality: It is important to eat high quality food. Choose foods that have a high nutritional value—that is, foods that are low in fat and sugar and that still provide the vitamins, minerals, and other nutrients your body needs.

Quantity: Control the size and number of portions you consume. Many people tend to overeat. One reason for this tendency is that it takes up to thirty minutes for your brain to recognize that your stomach is full. If you tend to overeat, try slowing down when you eat. This will allow your brain the time it needs to let you know when you should stop eating.

Timing: When you eat is important, especially if you're trying to lose weight. Experts recommend that people who are looking to lose weight or increase their energy levels try eating smaller, more frequent meals. Eating more frequently throughout the day forces the body's digestive system to stay active for longer periods, and burns extra calories in the process. You should eat the same total amount of food in the course of a day; otherwise, you may end up taking in more calories than you need. No matter how often you eat, it is important not to eat large meals just before bedtime, since calories consumed before long sedentary periods tend to be stored as fat.

NATURAL FOODS AND CLEAN EATING

In addition to affecting your weight, the food choices you make may affect your general health. For example, some studies suggest that eating foods that have not been overly processed or artificially enhanced may strengthen your immune system and increase your energy levels. Other research indicates that hormones and antibiotics added to animal feed can end up in our bodies when we eat meat from those animals.

Concern over animal feed additives has led to the growing popularity of organic foods, which are grown without using artificial fertilizers, pesticides, and additives. Organic food can be purchased at supermarkets and some specialty grocery stores. If you wish to avoid artificially enhanced foods, look in the supermarket or specialty grocery store for foods that bear descriptions such as "organic," "free-range," or "wild-caught."

FOODS TO FUEL YOUR WORKOUT

No matter what their source, different nutrients supply your body with what it needs to accomplish different tasks. Therefore, it is important to develop your diet based on the type and duration of your workouts.

When you're cardio training, choose foods that your body can digest slowly to provide consistent energy throughout your workout. These types of foods should provide a steady level of energy during a training session. Proteins and complex carbohydrates are a good choice. Have a small snack like a teaspoon of peanut butter with a small apple or half a turkey sandwich on whole grain bread. Eat your snack one to two hours before your workout. If you are looking for a quick burst of energy, you can snack on a granola bar or a banana.

While strength training, your meals should consist of high levels of carbohydrates and protein. Meals of this sort give you the energy to lift weights at your highest capacity and provide the basic building blocks for additional muscle. Meals should focus on complex carbohydrates and contain enough calories so that your body is able to perform well during the entire workout. Avoid sugars and other simple carbohydrates because eating these can lead to energy crashes in the middle of a workout. Eat your meals 30 to 90 minutes before a workout. An example of a good pre-workout meal would be a bowl of steel-cut oats with vanilla soy milk and three egg whites. For a quick snack before working out have a low-fat shake or protein bar that also contains carbohydrates.

POST-TRAINING NUTRITION

Since working out leaves you depleted of nutrients, it is important to replenish these nutrients as quickly as possible. Without proper post-workout nutrition, you may fail to see the optimum results of your workout. Eating the right foods immediately after a hard exercise session can boost your metabolism and help your muscles recover and become stronger. Meals should be carbohydrate- and protein-rich, with very little fat since fat slows the digestion process. Post-training meals should be eaten immediately after completion of the workout, preferably within 20 minutes. This is especially true if you're weight training, because immediately after working out, the body is prepared to direct protein to repair the tiny tears in the muscle tissue that occur when you lift weights. The longer you wait to replenish nutrients, the less effective they are at reaching targeted muscles. It is also important to remember that during this period the body will often produce strong feelings of hunger. You need to resist the temptation to eat a large, heavy meal, though. Have a serving of low-fat chocolate milk right after you work out. Since liquids digest easily, this snack will be effective at delivering nutrients exactly when your body needs them.

NUTRITIONAL SUPPLEMENTS

Making healthy, intelligent food choices is the best way to get the nutrients your body needs. However, if you are unable to eat balanced meals because of time or other restrictions, you can consider including vitamins, minerals and other nutritional supplements in your diet. These nutritional enhancements can help your body work at its maximum potential.

VITAMINS AND MINERALS

Many people find that supplements help them perform beyond their accustomed level, allowing them to reach new levels of fitness. A few popular supplements are:

Multivitamins: These come in a variety of forms—tablets, capsules, powders, or liquids. Whatever the form, a single dose contains a combination of vitamins and minerals that are essential to your body's functions. Most experts agree that taking a multivitamin is an excellent way to maintain your health and fitness.

Creatine: This is a chemical produced naturally in the body that can help transfer energy to muscles. Creatine is also available as a supplement. It is commonly used by athletes looking to improve muscle performance during high intensity strength training workouts. Creatine is also used by individuals looking to gain muscle mass. Debate over whether creatine supplements are a good idea is ongoing; anyone considering using creatine should consult a doctor before supplementing a diet with this substance.

Glutamine: This is an amino acid that is essential in the body's production of proteins, the main component of muscle tissue. Protein is also a vital component of other types of tissues and is important in the proper functioning of the immune system. Glutamine is severely depleted during strength training, leaving the body susceptible to muscle deterioration and other health problems.

Omega 3: This is an essential fatty acid found naturally in fish and linseed oil. It helps the heart perform efficiently during long cardiovascular exercise routines and recover faster after vigorous strength training.

PROTEIN POWDERS AND NUTRITIONAL SHAKES

Protein supplements that come in the form of powders or shakes increase the amount of protein available to your body without adding any fat to your diet. Protein is the most important component for developing muscles. Consuming protein powders and shakes appears to have little risk of side effects. However, these preparations, especially in concentrated forms, can be high in sugar and therefore may lead to weight gain in the form of body fat.

ENERGY AND PERFORMANCE ENHANCERS

Usually in the form of a pill, gels or liquids, energy supplements and performance enhancers are over-the-counter products that contain caffeine and other stimulants to boost the heart rate. They are typically used in order to maximize energy output during workout sessions. Individuals who take energy enhancers may benefit from improved endurance, concentration and coordination. It's important to understand that the long-term benefits that come from the use of these products have not been fully researched. We do know, however, that using these supplements has serious risks. Using them may lead to dehydration and other serious health complications. These stimulants are also potentially habit forming; they also may be dangerous to individuals who are at risk for cardiovascular disease or high blood pressure. Individuals who have been sedentary for a long period should also be wary of using these products. Do not take any energy or performance enhancers without first consulting your doctor.

No nutritional supplement, however, can take the place of paying attention to what you eat, how much, and when. Only by taking your nutrition seriously can you make the most of your fitness regimen.

WATER AND FITNESS

Water is essential to survival. Water constitutes more than two thirds of the human body. In addition, water is crucial to all of your body's major functions. Without enough water, you cannot digest food or eliminate wastes properly. Deprived of water, your body will quickly shut down.

THE IMPORTANCE OF WATER AND FLUIDS

Drinking enough water is crucial if we are to perform our day-to-day tasks effectively. When you do not have enough water, symptoms of dehydration quickly develop. Signs of dehydration include headaches, difficulty concentrating, and fatigue. Under such conditions, being effective at work or at home becomes difficult or impossible.

The consequences of dehydration are serious. Prolonged dehydration can increase the risk of kidney stones, infections and other serious health problems. On the other hand, maintaining hydration can have tremendous benefits. Recent studies have shown that people who drink at least eight glasses of water a day can decrease their risk of developing colon, bladder, and even breast cancer.

WHEN TO DRINK

As important as staying well hydrated is, it's easy to forget to drink water until dehydration has already set in. Research has shown that the best time to drink water is before you feel thirsty. Physical signs like dry mouth and sensations of thirst often occur only after you are dehydrated.

Even when people remember to drink water, they often fail to drink enough. The amount of water required for each individual is determined by his or her weight and metabolism. A rule of thumb for calculating your water consumption needs is to take your weight in pounds and divide it in half. The resulting number is the number of ounces of water you should consume. For example, a 180-pound person should drink 90 ounces of water per day. Some experts, however, suggest drinking even more water. They say that on average, men should drink around 120 ounces of water per day, while women should have around 90 ounces. No matter what your ideal water consumption is, remember to increase your water intake in conditions such as high heat, high altitude, low humidity, or high activity level.

SOURCES OF HYDRATION

A number of liquids and solid foods can provide your body with the water it needs:

Water: Your body uses water most readily in its plain, unadulterated form. The bulk (80-90%) of your hydration should come from drinking plain water.

Beverages: Drinking non-caffeinated beverages such as fruit juices, sports drinks, and milk is a good way of maintaining your hydration. Herbal teas also work well. Just remember that many beverages also contain sugar, fat, or both, which can add unwanted calories to your diet.

Fruits and vegetables: These solid foods consist mainly of water and therefore are excellent for hydration. Individuals who eat a healthy amount of fruits and vegetables may receive up to 20 percent of their hydration from these solid foods.

Be wary of drinking caffeinated beverages, such as coffee, tea and many soft drinks. Caffeine is a diuretic, meaning that it stimulates your kidneys to remove water from your system. If you feel the need for a caffeinated beverage, remember to compensate by drinking extra water.

HYDRATION BEFORE, DURING AND AFTER YOUR WORKOUT

Proper hydration is one of the easiest and most effective ways of boosting workout performance. Water is necessary in order for metabolism to take place, so being properly hydrated helps your body turn food into the energy you need for exercising. Water also helps your body regulate its temperature through sweating. Because vigorous exercise causes you to lose large amounts of water through sweating, it is important to drink water before, during, and after each workout session.

Pre-workout: Drink between 8 and 16 ounces of water in the hour prior to working out.

During workout: Replenish fluids by drinking 4 to 8 ounces of water every fifteen minutes. During vigorous cardiovascular training, or if you're exercising in hot temperatures, increase your water consumption in order to replace water lost from sweating.

After workout: Drink between 8 and 16 ounces of water within thirty minutes of completing your exercise routine. Your muscles need water in order to recover from the stress of a workout. Drinking proper amounts of water after your workout will help reduce muscle soreness and help you feel less tired.

Experts say that if your goal is to lose weight, you should increase the amount of water you consume before and after working out. Water is necessary for metabolism to take place. By keeping well hydrated, you will help your body burn calories.

DEHYDRATION AND POOR PERFORMANCE

Just as keeping hydrated enhances physical performance, dehydration leads to decreases in physical and mental performance. When you are dehydrated your body is unable to handle the physical exertions related to cardiovascular or strength exercises. As you become dehydrated, your blood volume can actually drop. A reduction in blood volume causes less oxygen to reach muscles, resulting in fatigue and loss of coordination. Your brain's oxygen supply is also reduced, leading to reduced concentration. Allowed to continue, dehydration can cause dizziness and loss of consciousness.

As you work to increase your level of fitness, keep in mind that an effective workout regimen depends largely on your ability to avoid fatigue and stay focused. Keeping well hydrated will allow you to just that.

PART 4: OPTIMIZING YOUR DIET TO MAXIMIZE YOUR RESULTS

The name of the person who first said, "You are what you eat" has long been lost to history, but those words are still true. What you eat directly affects your fitness. If you're trying to lose weight, you'll reach your goal much more easily if you adopt a sensible diet that reduces your caloric intake while maintaining a balanced nutrition. Similarly, if you're trying to build strength and muscle mass, your diet needs to reflect that goal. By eating the right foods in the right amounts, you can give yourself a huge boost toward meeting your fitness goals.

EATING TO LOSE WEIGHT

You lose weight when your body uses more energy than it consumes. Regular exercise and proper nutrition will help your body build muscle mass and increase your metabolism. This will help you lose weight faster and look trimmer. This chapter includes some basic guidelines that you can follow to help you burn fat, build muscle, and lose weight.

HEALTHY EATING

The food you eat provides your body with fuel. By eating healthy meals that provide the body with a mix of protein, carbohydrates, and fats, you will raise your metabolism and gain energy. An improper diet will decrease metabolism and leave you with less energy.

To lose weight, therefore, it is essential that you maintain a diet that includes all food groups in the right proportions. By emphasizing certain foods, such as lean meats and whole grains, you can encourage your body to burn more calories, resulting in faster weight loss. Lean meats like fish and turkey encourage the building of muscle. At the same time, these foods take longer to digest, helping you feel full longer. Whole grains have been shown to improve the body's digestion and boost metabolism. Your diet can include healthy fats, such as olive and canola oil, but avoid overindulgence in fats of any kind because it may lead you to gain weight.

HEALTHY SNACKING

Studies show that eating healthy snacks can help promote weight loss. If you wait until you're feeling famished before you eat, you may eat too much of the wrong foods. By keeping healthy snacks in your house and workplace, you can avoid the temptation to eat chips, cookies, and other unhealthy foods. When you buy snack foods, choose those that are both nutritious and low in calories. Limit your snacks to 200 calories or less. Here are a few suggestions for healthy snacks:

- Fruit, nuts, low-fat cheese or yogurt
- A slice of whole wheat bread and a teaspoon of peanut butter
- Turkey with vegetables on a half-round of pita bread
- Hard-boiled egg whites filled with hummus

ALTERNATIVES TO HIGH-CALORIE FOODS

In order to maintain a healthy diet it is important to plan and learn how to find healthier alternatives to satisfy high calorie cravings. Your new, healthy diet will leave you with more energy and fewer cravings. However, it is important to allow yourself the occasional treat. Food should be enjoyed, but only in proper moderation. If you have a history of over indulging in sweet or salty food you should pay close attention to the amount and frequency you indulge. For some individuals certain foods can trigger binge eating; these people may be better off avoiding these food triggers entirely.

High Calorie Craving and Low Calorie Solution

HIGH CALORIE CRAVINGS	LOW CALORIE SOLUTIONS
Potato Chips	Soy Crisps, Popcorn (air popped or low-fat microwave)
Candy, Candy Bars	Dried Fruit, Protein Bar (under 250 cal, less than 8 gms of fat)
Cake, Cookies, Pasteries	Whole grain cereal with skim milk and fruit
Ice Cream	Frozen berries blended with yogurt
Salty/Sweet	All nautral peanut butter with a banana
Chocolate	Dark Chocolate

WHEN TO EAT

Successful dieting requires planning. Take into consideration your eating habits to plan regular meals that include proper nutrition while controlling your caloric intake. The secret to losing weight and getting fit is to eat at regular intervals, rather than alternately starving and stuffing yourself.

Always eat breakfast. Studies have shown that those who enjoy a healthy breakfast are less likely to succumb to the kind of midday hunger that results in overeating. A proper breakfast, one that includes protein and complex carbohydrates, will give you energy that lasts throughout the day. Those who eat a healthy breakfast (one that includes both lean protein and carbohydrates) will consume fewer calories throughout the day than someone who skips breakfast. If you have high cholesterol or are looking for a healthy alternative to eggs, you can try an egg substitute or eat just the egg whites.

Make sure your meals are scheduled for approximately the same time every day. The body has a natural daily cycle that is crucial to appetite. By constantly switching your meal schedule, you will confuse your body, causing it to signal your brain that it needs food when it really doesn't. In addition, maintaining a regular eating schedule will help your body digest food properly.

Eat every three hours to prevent hunger and maintain energy levels. If you wait longer, your body will react by telling your brain that it needs food. The result will be increased hunger. By eating every three hours, you will feel more satisfied and full on less food.

Food needs time to be converted into calories and burned off, so it's a good idea to eat larger meals in the early part of the day. Large dinners eaten close to going to sleep will not be properly metabolized. During sleep your body is in resting mode; metabolism slows and excess calories are stored as fat.

TIPS TO HELP YOU LOSE WEIGHT

Here are a few tips to help you lose weight:

Increase fiber: This will help decrease hunger sensations and allow you to feel full longer. Studies show that fiber helps food to be efficiently digested and processed. Recent studies have also shown that increasing fiber in your diet may decrease your risk of colon cancer.

Stay hydrated: Water is essential to every bodily function. The more water you drink, the better the body functions and the more effectively it burns calories. Thirst can also be mistaken for hunger. If you've recently eaten and start to feel hungry, try drinking a glass of water instead of eating a snack.

Strength train: Muscles use more energy than other kinds of tissues. By building muscles through strength training, you will increase your body's overall metabolism and its ability to burn calories. It is especially important to strength train when you're dieting in order to maintain muscle mass.

Don't skip meals: Skipping meals or eating too little at a meal can be as harmful to your weight-loss goals as overeating. If you skip meals or eat too little, your metabolism will slow, making it harder to lose weight.

Eat metabolism-boosting foods: Eat fruits, vegetables and whole grains. These foods will help keep insulin levels steady so that you'll be able to metabolize food more efficiently. Foods like these also boost the efficiency of your digestive tract.

Get enough sleep: If you do not get adequate rest, your body attempts to compensate for low energy levels by creating cravings for sugar and other simple carbohydrates. Sleep allows your body to recover from vigorous exercise, making it easier for you to stay active without resorting to eating high-calorie foods.

Eat slower: Studies show that it can take as long as half an hour for your brain to realize that your stomach is full. By eating more slowly, you'll probably feel satisfied on less food.

Avoid high-fat food preparation: Prepare foods in a healthy way. Avoid cooking with oil (e.g. frying, sautéing, deep frying); instead, try recipes that call for grilling, poaching, or baking.

Eat out sensibly: Avoid foods like bread and chips, which provide calories but no real nutrition. Order a soup or salad instead of an appetizer. This will help you avoid high-calorie foods that don't satisfy your appetite. Be aware of the size of the entrée and consider taking part of it home. Often, single portions served at most restaurants are large enough for two or even three meals.

AVOIDING WEIGHT LOSS FAILURE

The most common reason people fail to lose weight is that they forget commonsense dietary rules. We often become over-zealous in our attempts to lose weight or forget that there are no shortcuts to losing weight. Resorting to crash diets and similar desperate measures will often lead to increases, not decreases, in weight. Here are some of the common ways that dieters end up sabotaging their attempts to lose weight:

Skipping meals: Often, individuals who skip meals become so hungry that they end up overeating. Going without eating encourages a negative attitude towards food as something to be denied, rather than a normal part of a healthy lifestyle.

A diet too low in calories: With too few calories, the body goes into starvation mode, slowing the metabolism and storing energy in the form of fat.

Low carbohydrate diet: Severely limiting carbohydrates reduces your body's ability to metabolize food properly. Carbohydrates are the body's main source of energy, and foods like bread and pasta contain vitamins that help your body burn calories efficiently. People on low-carbohydrate diets often experience diminished results after rapid initial weight-loss.

Eliminating too much fat: Denying your body the amount of fat it needs keeps it from making use of essential nutrients, such as vitamins A, D, E, and K, which are fat-soluble.

Too little protein: Protein is essential to the construction and maintenance of lean muscle. Decreasing your body's intake of protein keeps you from building muscle mass, resulting in a slowing of your metabolism. Remember: Muscles burn more calories than other tissues, whether the body is active or at rest. If your muscle mass decreases, so will your burning of calories.

Too much alcohol: Because alcohol is easily converted to fat, consuming beer, wine, or liquor makes losing weight much more difficult.

Processed foods: Processed foods like chips and some meats can be high in fat. Eating these (or any high-fat food) adds calories without making you feel full.

Too many "diet foods": Do not substitute diet foods for substantial meals. High-calorie breakfast drinks, for example, do little to fill you up, meaning that you're more likely to overeat at lunch. This will hinder your overall weight loss.

Low-fat/high-sugar food: Although some foods are labeled as "low-fat," they are often high in sugar. A large infusion of sugar will cause a spike in your blood sugar levels. While you will feel energized for a short period of time, the subsequent sugar "crash" will lead to more food cravings.

The following table suggests a diet that will promote, rather than hinder, weight-loss:

Sample Diet for Weight Loss

SAMPLE DIET FOR IMPROVED ENERGY

Meal	Sunday	Monday	Tuesday	Wednesday	Thursday	Friday	Saturday
Breakfast	Egg white omelet Multivitamin	Bran muffin & 1/2 grapefruit Multivitamin	Whole wheat cereal with non-fat milk Multivitamin	Whole wheat pancakes with fruit Multivitamin	Oatmeal Multivitamin	Yogurt with granola Multivitamin	Egg white omelet Multivitamin
Mid Morning Snack	Whole grain cereal with non-fat milk	Boiled egg	Banana	Cereal bar	Whole grain bread with natural peanut butter	Carrots and celery sticks	Pear
Lunch	Turkey sandwich on whole wheat no mayo	Salad with low fat dressing	Chicken vegetable soup	Turkey sandwich on whole wheat no mayo	Minestrone soup	Turkey sandwich on whole wheat no mayo	Salad with low fat dressing
Afternoon Snack	Dried apricots	Protein bar	Turkey and veggies in 1/2 whole wheat pita	Soy chips	Popcorn	Cottage cheese (low fat)	Veggies
Dinner	Grilled chicken breast salad	Soy burger with side salad	Grilled salmon with asparagus	Soup & salad with low fat dressing	Grilled chicken fajitas	Whole wheat pasta with meat sauce	Baked stuffed eggplant
Evening Snack	popcorn	1/2 cup of mixed nuts (without salt)	Apple	Yogurt with fruit	Dark chocolate	Strawberries	Apple with 1/2 cup of cashews

EATING TO INCREASE
STRENGTH AND MUSCLE MASS

In order to increase your strength and muscle mass, it is essential that you eat the proper foods. Your body needs carbohydrates so it has energy for training, and it needs protein so it can build muscle mass. As you exercise more, you will need to consume more calories, but this should not be seen as a license to overindulge in sweets or other junk foods. The food you eat should be chosen to provide both energy and nutrients.

WHAT YOU SHOULD EAT

When you're attempting to increase strength and muscle mass, you'll need to increase your intake of complex carbohydrates and lean protein. At the same time, it is important to maintain a balanced diet. That means you'll still need to consume sensible amounts of fats and even some simple carbohydrates.

Carbohydrates are your primary source of energy. This energy is used to support the rigorous training that will lead to increased muscle mass. Lack of sufficient carbohydrates can hinder training in two ways. First, the lack of calories can lead to physical and mental fatigue. You may not be able to work as hard or for as long as you would if your energy levels were high. Second, if you don't consume enough carbohydrates, your body will be forced to burn protein it would otherwise use for building muscle. If you continue to deprive it of carbohydrates, your body will eventually start consuming whatever muscle tissue you already have. Your body may, essentially, end up breaking down the very muscle you are trying to build up.

Traditionally, diets designed to help increase muscle mass have called for consuming high amounts of protein. However, you should avoid eating too much protein. If your goal is to gain muscle, you should generally aim for consuming 1.2 – 2 grams of protein per each pound of body weight. Many high-protein diets involve exceeding this guideline, but if you do so, you are just consuming calories that will probably be turned into fat.

When your goal is building strength, it is important to avoid foods that are high in fat or sugar. Eating these foods will slow the development of muscle mass because you will be filling up on them instead of nutrient-rich foods. It's important to limit your intake of fat. Although fat is essential to your body's functioning, eating large quantities of fat can cause you to gain weight without adding muscle. It is also important to avoid sugars, alcohol and refined white flour. These calorie-rich foods often lead to spikes in your blood sugar and a subsequent feeling of sluggishness and fatigue.

TIMING YOUR MEALS

In trying to build muscle mass, when you eat is just as important as what you eat. Experts recommend that you eat carbohydrates before you train and plenty of protein after you train. Make sure you eat complex carbohydrates before you lift weights. This will not only give you sufficient energy to exercise properly, but will prepare your body to repair and build new muscle tissue after you've worked out. When you consume carbohydrates, insulin levels in your bloodstream rise. Insulin plays a key role in bringing the amino acids that make up protein into the muscles. So by consuming the proper balance of carbohydrates and proteins at the right time, you'll be able to repair and build muscle tissue faster.

Sample Diet for Weight Training

SAMPLE DIET FOR IMPROVED ENERGY

Meal	Sunday	Monday	Tuesday	Wednesday	Thursday	Friday	Saturday
Breakfast	Egg white omelet Multivitamin	Bran muffin, grapefruit, turkey sausage Multivitamin	Whole wheat cereal with nonfat milk Multivitamin	Oatmeal Multivitamin	Bran muffin, grapefruit, turkey sausage Multivitamin	Whole wheat cereal wit nonfat milk Multivitamin	Egg white omelet Multivitamin
Mid Morning Snack	Whole grain cereal with non-fat milk	Boiled egg	Banana and low fat string cheese	Protein bar	Whole grain bread with natural peanut butter	Yogurt with granola	Protein bar
Lunch	Turkey sandwich on whole wheat no mayo	Turkey breast salad with low fat dressing	Soy burger	Chicken vegetable soup & small salad	Grilled chicken breast with veggies	Turkey sandwich on whole wheat no mayo	Beef stew (low fat & low sodium)
Afternoon Snack	Popcorn	Protein bar	Turkey jerky	Soy chips	Cottage cheese (low fat)	Protein Bar	Turkey and veggies in 1/2 whole wheat pita
Dinner	Grilled fish	Whole wheat pasta with meat sauce	Grilled chicken fajitas	BBQ chicken grilled with corn	Turkey with mash potatoes & peas	Grilled chicken breast salad	Grilled salmon with asparagus
Evening Snack	1/2 cup of mixed nuts (without salt)	Yogurt with fruit	Popcorn	Apple with 1/2 cup of cashews	Dark chocolate	Yogurt with granola	Popcorn

EATING TO IMPROVE

ENERGY LEVELS

Without sufficient energy to work out, you will be unable to increase fitness. If you do not eat the right foods, fail to eat properly before or after training, or limit calories in the interests of weight loss, you'll lack the energy to get through your workouts. If you are adding physical training to your daily routine, you have to increase your food intake to provide your body the energy it needs. If you constantly feel tired or experience "heavy legs" during your warm up and can't quite pick up your feet, chances are you simply need to eat. Consuming carbohydrates should make you feel better.

WHAT YOU SHOULD EAT

Anyone who is looking to improve their energy level should maintain a diet that meets the daily nutritional requirements published by the federal government. Such a diet means avoiding eating sweets and processed foods, which are often high in salt, sugar, and fat. Meals should concentrate on complex carbohydrates, such as whole-grain breads and cereals. These foods are digested more slowly by the body than simple carbohydrates are, and help promote steady blood sugar levels. Drink ample amounts of water and avoid food that is fried or prepared with excessive fat or butter.

Just as you can boost your energy level by eating right, other practices can sap your body of energy. Here are some things to avoid:

Excess caffeine: Often people looking for a quick burst of energy will turn to caffeine; however, this often has the opposite effect. Although caffeine is a stimulant, once it's eliminated from your body it can leave you feeling weak and tired. In addition, more than 2 cups of a caffeinated drink per day can interfere with sleep, making you feel even more fatigued.

Large, high-calorie meals: If you overeat before exercising, your body focuses on digesting food. Digestion requires a large amount of blood flow to your stomach and intestines, meaning there's less blood available to carry oxygen to your muscles.

Sodas and junk food: These are loaded with simple carbohydrates that are quickly digested, resulting in high blood sugar levels. Although you may feel an initial burst of energy as your blood sugar levels spike, that energy burst is quickly followed by sluggishness and fatigue. In addition, your body can turn excess sugar into fat, leaving you heavier without contributing to strength and fitness.

Sample Diet for Improved Energy

SAMPLE DIET FOR IMPROVED ENERGY

Meal	Sunday	Monday	Tuesday	Wednesday	Thursday	Friday	Saturday
Breakfast	Oatmeal Multivitamin	Whole wheat bagel with low fat cream cheese Multivitamin	Egg white omelet Multivitamin	Bran muffin, 1/2 grapefruit, Multivitamin	Oatmeal Multivitamin	Whole wheat cereal with nonfat milk Multivitamin	Whole wheat bagel with low fat cream cheese & lox Multivitamin
Mid Morning snack	Raw veggies	Dried cranberries	Banana	Carrot and celery sticks	Whole grain bread with natural peanut butter	Yogurt	Cereal Bar
Lunch	Grilled chicken breast salad	Clam chowder soup	Turkey sandwich on whole wheat no mayo	Vegetable soup	Salad with low fat dressing	Soy burger	Natural peanut butter sandwich on whole wheat
Afternoon Snack	Apple with 1/2 cup of cashews	Celery with natural peanut butter	Soy chips	Cottage cheese (low fat)	Popcorn	Protein Bar	Banana
Dinner	Turkey and veggies in whole wheat pita	Grilled chicken breast with steamed broccoli	Grilled portobello mushroom with whole grain rice	Grilled salmon with asparagus	Whole wheat pasta with meat sauce	Turkey vegetable soup with garden salad	Shrimp, veggies and pineapple shish kabob
Evening Snack	Dark chocolate	Dried apricots	Popcorn	Yogurt with fruit	Dark chocolate	1/2 cup of mixed nuts (without salt)	Dried cherries

PART 5: WORKOUT PRODUCTS AND SERVICES

Even before you start your journey to fitness, you've got some decisions to make. For one thing, you must decide where you'll go for your workouts. Will you go to a gym or train at home? Will you work alone with a personal trainer or join a class? Before you begin your first workout, of course, you'll have to have the right clothing and equipment. Dressing appropriately will help you feel more comfortable during your workouts. The right equipment will help you make the most of the time you spend working out.

OPTIONS FOR WORKING OUT

There are four primary options to choose from when creating your workout program: (1) Gym, (2) Personal trainer, (3) Training at home, and (4) Group training. Each of these choices has both benefits and disadvantages. Examine your personal fitness goals and personal preferences before selecting the option that is right for you.

GYM MEMBERSHIP

Gyms offer a large selection of equipment for strength, cardiovascular and flexibility training. Gyms come in many forms. Some are owned by national chains and offer memberships for a monthly fee. Others are operated by a local educational institution, such as a college or university, and may make memberships available to those who live in the local community. Depending on the size of your community, there may be a gym operated by a non-profit organization like the YMCA or Boys and Girls Club.

When looking for a gym, examine its proximity to your home and workplace as well as the hours of operation and the amenities the gym provides. Don't downplay the importance of a gym's hours and amenities. If the place is closed at the times you can work out, or if the locker rooms make you queasy because they smell bad, you're not likely to benefit from your membership. Most gyms will allow prospective members to work out a few times as a trial for free or a nominal fee. Visit the gym at the time you expect to go normally and see if you feel comfortable there. If possible, meet with the staff members who lead classes that you might want to take. The following table will help you weigh the advantages and disadvantages of joining a gym.

Pros and Cons of a Gym Membership

PROS	CONS
Workout year round unaffected by the weather	Must travel to and from gym adding time to workout
Variety - Cardio, machines, free weights and strtching facilities	Cost - Gym memberships can be expensive
Higher quality equipment maintained by professionals	Requires proper training on equipment - machines are complex

PERSONAL TRAINING

Working out with a personal trainer is an excellent way to get fit. A trainer will help motivate you through difficult times and help you maximize your workout sessions. Trainers typically schedule hour-long workouts from one to three times a week. Because a trainer knows just when to increase the rigor of your workouts, you will reach your goals faster than you would on your own. A trainer will help you track your progress and will alter your fitness routine as your needs change. It is important to find a trainer you like. Make sure the trainer you hire is both knowledgeable and properly certified.

Pros and Cons of Personal Trainers

PROS	CONS
Excellent motivation, guidance and support. External enforcer always encouraging you to push harder	Very expensive - Often you have to join a gym & pay for sessions on top of membership fees
Expertise - A trainer will help explain and illustrate proper technique	Time constraints - You have to work out during set sessions.
	Expense - Sessions usually come in groups and often cannot be refunded even if you miss a session.

AT HOME

Fitness can easily be achieved even if you do not choose to join a gym or hire a personal trainer. Individual sports such as running, hiking, and bicycling can be excellent forms of cardiovascular training. With the purchase of a treadmill, elliptical trainer, or workout video, you can work out indoors, year-round.

Many prefer the comfort and privacy of working out at home. However, working out at home requires more self-discipline than the other options do. Your home is full of distractions. It's easy to succumb to the temptation to do household chores or sit in front of the TV, especially if you've had a long day at work.

If you want to work out in your own home, a few additional pieces of equipment will help you train effectively on your own. There are various fitness solutions for strength training at home. Your options range from simple hand weights and resistance bands to large home gyms with stationary bikes and weight machines. Select a system that meets your needs. Keep in mind the available space in your home. Then consider the expense of the equipment. You may end up deciding that a membership at a gym is a better choice. The following table will help you decide if training at home is right for you.

Pros and Cons of at Home Training

PROS	CONS
Exercise at your own convenience.	Distractions - work, family TV
Train periodically during the day as your schedule allows	Limited options - especially in regard to strength training, risk of injury
Inexpensive	Lack of external motivation
	Outdoor activities limited by weather

GROUP EXERCISE

Group exercise is any type of fitness class in which an instructor leads all the participants through a series of exercise routines. Classes are usually held in a large room and can include aerobic exercises, strength training, flexibility training, or any combination of these. Classes are usually one hour long and include warm-up and cool-down routines. Exercises may or may not be set to music. Group exercise can be a great way to fulfill all of your fitness requirements for cardio, strength, and flexibility training. With the variety of classes that are available today, you are sure to find a class that suits your needs and is appropriate for your level of fitness.

Most gyms offer a selection of group exercise classes that are either free to members or require only a small additional charge. Dance studios often offer fitness classes that are available to anyone for a per-class fee. Private studios that focus on specific types of exercises such as pilates, yoga, kick boxing, and aerobics usually offer group classes. These studios usually offer packages that include a series of sessions at a reduced rate or a single session for a higher rate.

Most gyms and studios offer a set number of classes that may or may not work with your schedule. Check the availability of classes in your area. Choose times that do not conflict with other commitments to ensure that you don't have any excuses not to attend. Classes have limited space and often are on a first come, first served basis. If you do not arrive to your class on time, chances are that the class may have reached capacity. Some classes have a sign up sheet where you can sign in 30 min in advance to guarantee your spot.

Pros and Cons of Group Exercise

PROS	CONS
Instructor, as well as other participants motivate you through your workout	If you have never participated in group exercise, classes may seem intimidating. Start with a beginning class.
Set class schedules means you have to commit ahead of time and plan to workout	If classes are cancelled or switched, you will miss your workout unless you are prepared to workout on your own. If you are traveling or out of town, you will ned to find an alternative to your usual workout

CLOTHING AND ACCESSORIES

Before you get started on your journey to fitness, here are several helpful guidelines that will help you achieve your goals.

CLOTHING AND SHOES

Always make sure your clothes are appropriate for the activity you are engaging in. Select clothes made from material that "breathes" and that will not constrict your movements. If you're planning to exercise outdoors, be certain your clothes are appropriate for the weather.

Shoes are more important than any other article of clothing. Choose shoes that offer support and proper cushioning. In order to avoid injury and sore muscles, it is essential to have shoes that fit properly. You should have half an inch of space between the front of the shoe and your longest toe. Walk around, run in place and jump up and down to check the fit. Your heel should not move around. Good shoes that fit properly should be comfortable right away. Never purchase athletic shoes with the idea that they are going to get more comfortable after you break them in.

Replace shoes if you experience any aches and pains in your feet, knees, legs, and hips or lower back. It is important to replace shoes that are worn out. Running shoes should be replaced after 4 to 6 months; shoes used for workout classes should be replaced once a year. Purchase shoes through a store where the sales clerks understand your needs and can measure your feet properly.

FITNESS ACCESSORIES

It is important to have the proper fitness accessories to help maximize performance and promote a happy workout experience.

Music: For many people, music is essential for working out. Music from a portable MP3 player, radio, or CD player can help motivate you and keep your pace steady.

Pedometer or Heart Monitor: A pedometer can help you keep track of the distance you run or walk; a heart monitor can help you tailor your workout to enhance cardiac conditioning. These devices can be used to help you set new goals for future workouts as well.

Gym bag: It is important to have a bag that is dedicated for trips to the gym. A proper bag will hold all your fitness equipment and have room for clothes to change into after working out.

Water bottle: By carrying a water bottle while you work out, you will be able to stay hydrated without having to interrupt your session to visit the water fountain.

PREVENT INJURIES

You can avoid many injuries by knowing your limitations and by taking all necessary precautions before working out. Never overexert yourself. Learn proper techniques and form before performing exercises with large amounts of weight. Pace yourself and work with a partner or spotter when training with heavy free weights.

No matter what kind of workout you choose, proper preparation will enable you to make the most of your available time and maximize your efforts to get fit.

PART 6: PERSONAL DATA

In order to measure the success of your fitness program, it's important to establish your starting point. Filling out the worksheets in this section will help you do just that. Take the time to answer each question as completely and accurately as you can. The data you provide in these worksheets will also help you identify fitness and nutritional issues that need special attention.

NOTES

YOUR FITNESS AND NUTRITION

PROFILE

This chapter includes a series of worksheets that will help you ascertain your current fitness and nutritional profile. These worksheets will also be used as a baseline so that you can measure your progress. Take the time to fill out each worksheet. Be honest and accurate with your responses. Since you should consult your healthcare provider before starting a new fitness program, you can ask him or her for any information you don't already have at hand.

Worksheet: Your Personal Health Profile

Name: _____

Date: _____

MEASUREMENTS	INITIAL	3 MONTHS	6 MONTHS	9 MONTHS	12 MONTHS
Weight					
Body Fat %					
BMI					
Total Cholesterol					
HDL Cholesteral					
LDL Cholesteral					
Blood Pressure					
Glucose					
Physical Activity	mins/day				
Smoking	per day				
Alcoholic Drinks	per week				

Other:

_____

_____

_____

WORKSHEET: NUTRITIONAL WORKSHEET

Nutrition Worksheet

Name: _____

Date: _____

TEST	INITIAL	3 MONTHS	6 MONTHS	9 MONTHS	12 MONTHS
Meals	per day				
Breakfast	per week				
Meals Skipped	per week				
Late Meals	per week				
Fast Food Meals	per week				
Fried Foods	per serving				
Fruits/Vegetables	per day				
Glasses of Water	per day				
Caffeine	per day				
Multivitamin	daily dosage				

WORKSHEET: PHYSICAL ACTIVITY READINESS QUESTIONNAIRE (PAR-Q)

It is important to make sure your body is in proper working order before beginning any fitness routine. Take a moment to go through the following checklist. If you answer yes to any of the following questions, please see a medical professional.

Have you ever been told by a medical professional that you have a heart condition?

_____

_____

Do you feel pain in your chest during physical activity?

_____

_____

Have you experienced chest pain in the last month when not engaged in strenuous physical activity?

Have you ever lost consciousness or lost your balance because you became dizzy while engaging in physical activity?

Have you ever lost your balance or lost consciousness when not undergoing physical activity?

Do you suffer from joint or bone ailments or injuries that could be exacerbated by physical activity?

Are you taking prescription drugs for high blood pressure or any heart condition?

Do you know of any other reason why you should not engage in physical activity?

FITNESS HISTORY

At what age were you in your best physical shape?

Have you ever participated in a workout program?

When?

How long did you stay with the program?

What did the program include?

What lead you to or inspired you to get into shape now?

What obstacles have kept you from meeting your previous fitness goals?

What will ensure these obstacles do not inhibit you this time?

Rate your current fitness level on a scale of 1-10 (1=Worst 10=Best)?

YOUR FITNESS GOALS

By first identifying your goals, you can create a specific workout routine to help you achieve them. Your goals should be specific, quantifiable, realistic and time-based. Fill out the following surveys honestly and with a critical eye. You'll be able to use the resulting information to inspire yourself and ward off possible fitness pitfalls.

FITNESS PREFERENCES

What do you want to accomplish with your workout program?

(Check the boxes next to the goals that are most important to you.)

- ☐ Improve cardiovascular fitness/endurance
- ☐ Improve diet/eating habits
- ☐ Improve flexibility
- ☐ Improve health
- ☐ Improve strength
- ☐ Improve muscle tone & shape
- ☐ Increase energy
- ☐ Gain weight
- ☐ Lose weight
- ☐ Prevent injury/Rehabilitate injury
- ☐ Reduce cholesterol
- ☐ Reduce blood pressure
- ☐ Reduce risk of disease
- ☐ Reduce stress
- ☐ Train for a sports-specific event
- ☐ Other: _____

What types of physical activity do you enjoy and why?

_____

_____

What types of physical activity do you dislike and why?

Do you prefer to exercise alone, with a partner, or in a group? Why?

Exercise Excuses/Solutions Questionnaire

EXCUSES	SOLUTIONS
I can't exercise because I'm too tired	I'll workout for 5 minutes & see if I'm still tired ·
I can't exercise because the gym is too far away	I'll workout at home, maybe go for a walk or do a fitness DVD
I can't exercise because I'm too sore	I'll focus on my stretching, by stretching I will help alleviate soreness and decrease the chances of further injury.
I can't exercise because I'm embarrassed about my body	That's the best reason to workout, not working out will leave your mind time to worry and wallow.
I can't exercise because I'm embarrassed about my body	Play with your kids, playing sports with your children will give an opportunity to bond with them over something they enjoy
I can't exercise because...	
I can't exercise because...	
I can't exercise because...	
I can't exercise because...	
I can't exercise because...	

WORKSHEET: WORKOUT PLAN QUESTIONNAIRE

A successful workout plan is one that includes activities you enjoy. Be honest in answering the following questions and you will be able to develop a plan you can maintain.

Which types of physical activity do you enjoy participating in?

Aerobics	Martial arts
Active gardening	Pilates
Backpacking	Racquetball/handball
Baseball/softball	Roller blading
Bicycling/spinning	Rowing
Climbing	Soccer
Cross country skiing	Skating
Dancing	Stair/bench stepping
Downhill skiing	Stretching
Football	Swimming
Golfing	Tennis
Hiking	Volleyball
Hockey	Walking
Jogging/running	Weight training
Jump roping	Yoga

What type of clothes will these activities require?

Shoes?

Specialty Clothes?

Specialty Equipment?

Miscellaneous?

How many times a week do you want to workout?
　　1-2 days
　　2-3 days
　　3-4 days
　　5+ days

How long will each session be?
　　10-20 minutes
　　20-30 minutes
　　30-40 minutes
　　50 + minutes

What days of the week do you have available for exercising?
_____

_____

How will you warm-up and cool down for each workout?
_____

_____

What is your secondary plan if your original workout plan doesn't work?
_____

_____

If exercising outside, do you have a contingency plan for bad weather?
_____

How will you measure your progress?
_____

_____

How long do you think it will take to reach your goal?
_____

_____

YOUR WORKOUT SCHEDULE

When creating your workout schedule, consider what you are trying to achieve. Your goals will determine the type of activity, intensity, frequency, and duration of your workouts. If your goal is to lose weight, you will probably want to focus on cardiovascular activities, while those looking to gain weight and build muscle mass will need to focus on weight training. Review your fitness goals questionnaire and pinpoint the main goals. That way you can tailor your program to achieve the maximum results. Take into account your age, current health and fitness level, personal interests, and schedule.

As you develop your workout program, remember that it should include all three components of fitness: cardiovascular conditioning, strength, and flexibility. Training in all three areas will improve your performance in your target area while enhancing your overall fitness. Another important aspect of each workout session is proper warm-up and cool-down activities. Be sure to include both of these in your program.

As you schedule your workouts for each week, be sure to take one day to rest. It's just as important to allow your body to recover and rebuild as it is to train hard. If you don't allow proper time for your body to heal and recuperate, you will slow your progress and may never reach your goals.

If you are still unsure of where to begin, below are some activities that you should include in your workout program. You can modify this program gradually as your endurance, strength and skill levels improve.

Warm-up: 5-10 minutes of low intensity/low impact exercise such as walking, slow jogging, knee lifts, arm circles or trunk rotations.

Strength training: Aim for at least two 30-minute sessions per week that may include free weights, weight machines, resistance equipment, muscular endurance training and toning activities such as power yoga or pilates. Be sure to include activities that exercise each of the major muscle groups in these sessions.

Cardiovascular training: Participate in a 30-minute session of aerobic activity at least three times a week. You want to make sure the activity is continuous and is vigorous enough to require increased oxygen consumption. You should breathe hard, but not be so short of breath that you can't carry on a conversation. Typical activities include jogging/running, elliptical training, bicycling/spinning, cardio classes such as step aerobics, kick boxing, and aerobic dance.

Flexibility training: Do 10-15 minutes of stretching per day. An easy way to incorporate flexibility training is by stretching for several minutes after your warm-up and during your cool-down.

Cool-down: Expect to take 5-10 minutes to cool down after your session. Your cool-down can include slow walking or low intensity or low impact exercises with your stretching. Allow your heart rate, breathing and body temperature to gradually drop to normal levels. Use this time to relax and recover from your workout.

WORKSHEET: YOUR WORKOUT PROGRAM

Using what you have learned in this book, fill out the following worksheet to create your personalized workout program.

I. CARDIOVASCULAR TRAINING

Describe your cardiovascular training program:

_____

_____

_____

_____

How many training sessions do you plan per week?

_____

How long will each session last?

_____

II. STRENGTH TRAINING

Describe your strength training program?

_____

_____

_____

_____

How many training sessions do you plan per week?

_____

How long will each session last?

_____

III. FLEXIBILITY TRAINING

Describe your flexibility training program?

_____

_____

_____

_____

How many training sessions do you plan per week?

_____

How long will each session last?

_____

IV. WEEKLY WORKOUT PROGRAM AND SCHEDULE

Once you have completed the previous sections, fill out the following chart to create a weekly workout schedule for yourself to go with your workout program worksheet.

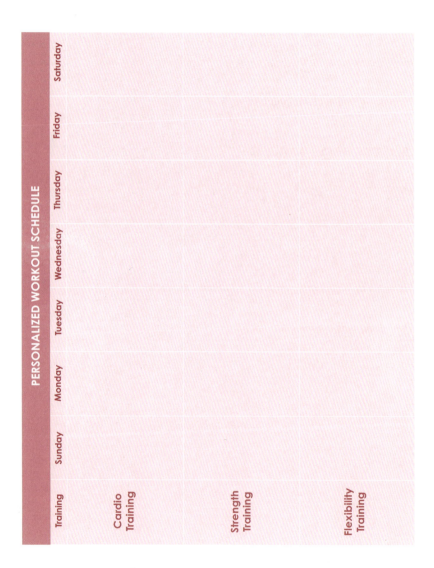

PERSONALIZED WORKOUT SCHEDULE

Training	Sunday	Monday	Tuesday	Wednesday	Thursday	Friday	Saturday
Cardio Training							
Strength Training							
Flexibility Training							

WORKSHEET: YOUR NUTRITIONAL PROGRAM

Using what you have learned in this book, fill out the following worksheet
to create your personalized nutritional program.

Describe your nutritional program:

What are your nutritional program goals?

How many calories will you consume daily?

How many meals will you have each day?

Will you take a multivitamin or supplements?

What is your target nutritional balance? (in grams)

	In Grams	% of daily recommended amount
Fat		
Protein		
Carbohydrate		
Fiber		

CREATING A PERSONALIZED MENU

Use the following table to create a personalized menu. Make copies of this table prior to using it. You will be able to design a menu plan for several months.

Create Your Menu: Week _____

Personalized Menu	Sunday	Monday	Tuesday	Wednesday	Thursday	Friday	Saturday
Meal							
Breakfast							
Mid Morning Snack							
Lunch							
Afternoon Snack							
Dinner							
Evening Snack							
Calories							

TRACKING YOUR RESULTS

Use the following worksheet to keep track of your progress over the next 12 months. Write down your initial measurements.

Initial Measurements

Date: _____   BMI: _____   Hips: _____

Weight: _____   Chest: _____   Thigh:_____

Body Fat %:_____   Waist: _____   Bicep:_____

MEASURE	MONTH 1	MONTH 2	MONTH 3	MONTH 4	MONTH 5	MONTH 6
Weight						
Body Fat %						
BMI						
Chest						
Waist						
Hips						
Thigh						
Bicep						

MEASURE	MONTH 7	MONTH 8	MONTH 9	MONTH 10	MONTH 11	MONTH 12
Weight						
Body Fat %						
BMI						
Chest						
Waist						
Hips						
Thigh						
Bicep						

Take an initial photo when you begin your workout program. In one month, take another photo place it below your initial photo. Continue replacing the "current photo" as you see progress on your physical appearance. Be proud of your success.

Place initial photo here.

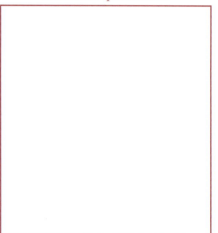

Place current photo here.

Change this picture as you see progress on your physical look.

PART 7: DAILY WORKOUT JOURNAL

To make the most of your workouts, you should keep track of your progress so that you can see yourself approaching your fitness goals. Keeping track of your progress on a daily and weekly basis is the best way to stay motivated and continue working on your fitness program. You can also quickly tell if your progress is slowing down and take action to get yourself back on track. The pages that follow will help you make the most of your fitness program.

GETTING STARTED

Take a moment each day to **weigh yourself**. For consistency, do this with no clothes and as soon as you wake up in the morning. Record your **energy level** as well. Read the **helpful tip** for each day. If that tip gives you any ideas for new exercises or modifications to your routine, write those down in the **workout reminder** section of the page.

CARDIOVASCULAR EXERCISE

Before you start working out do not forget to stretch or warm up. Record this in your journal. Make note of any exercise you do on that day to build cardiovascular fitness. Write down the time you start each exercise and how many minutes you spend on the exercise. Depending on the type of exercise, it may also be appropriate to note the distance involved. As much as possible, estimate the number of calories burned by each exercise. Be certain to jot down any comments you have at the end of your cardiovascular session. Did you feel any pain? Is it getting easier? Do you think it is time to increase the intensity or length of your work out time? What changes, if any, do you want to make?

STRENGTH TRAINING

Use a similar procedure for the strength training section. Note the exercises you do, the muscle group(s) each exercise focuses on, and the number of repetitions for each set. Be sure to note the target area for each strength training session—upper body, lower body, or abs. Write down any comments you might have.

GROUP EXERCISE

Write down the time you start a group exercise. A group exercise might consist of a yoga class, dancing, or some other activity. Write down what the class or group exercise consisted of and how long it lasted. As accurately as possible, calculate the calories you burned during the activity. Be sure to note whether or not you did any stretching or warm-up exercises before starting the group activity.

GOALS

At the end of each day write down your daily goals for the next day. You'll find a blank at the top of each right-hand page where you can do this. Be ambitious in setting your goals, but be realistic, too. Don't defeat yourself by setting goals you have no hope of achieving. When you set goals that challenge you but are achievable, every day presents an opportunity to celebrate success.

A few examples of daily goals could be to do 30 minutes of strength training and running 3 miles in 30 minutes, or stretching for 20 minutes and doing one hour of aerobic exercise. Another daily goal could be, do not drink any alcohol.

When you achieve your daily goal place a gold star (found in the front of the book) in the upper right hand corner.

FLEXIBILITY TRAINING

Make certain that you note the exercises you do to increase flexibility. Keep track of the time you spend on this very important aspect of fitness training. In the comments section, you can make a note of exercises that seemed particularly helpful, or perhaps ones that you need to concentrate on in the future.

NUTRITIONAL INTAKE

Because fitness depends on developing healthy eating habits, be sure to write down what you ate for breakfast, lunch, dinner, and between-meal snacks. Note how much of each food you ate, the number of calories you consumed, and the nutrition facts for each food. If you take vitamins or other dietary supplements, indicate how much of those you consume. It is also very important to keep track of how much water you drink.

COMMENTS

You'll find space to write down any comments you have regarding your workout. This is where you can record what went well with your exercise session, what didn't go so well, and how you feel about your progress.

DATE:_____ WEEK#:_____ DAY#:_____ WEIGHT:_____

Helpful Tips

Daily Workout Journal

Exercise can substantially reduce the risk of developing or dying from diabetes, colon cancer and obesity-related illnesses.

CARDIOVASCULAR EXERCISE   STRETCHING/WARMUP: yes ☐ no ☐

Time	Exercise Type	Minutes	Distance	Pace/ Setting	Cal. Burned
CARDIO EXERCISE TOTALS:					

COMMENTS:

STRENGTH TRAINING   TARGET AREA: upper body ☐ lower body ☐ abs ☐

Exercise Type	Muscle Group	SET 1 Reps/Wt.	SET 2 Reps/Wt.	SET 3 Reps/Wt.	SET 4 Reps/Wt.
STRENGTH TRAINING TOTALS:					

WORKOUT REMINDER:

COMMENTS:

OTHER · GROUP EXERCISE   STRETCHING/WARMUP: yes ☐ no ☐

Time	Exercise Type	Minutes	Cal. Burned
OTHER · GROUP EXERCISE TOTALS:			

COMMENTS:

DAILY GOAL(S) _____

_____

_____

**DAILY GOALS
ACHIEVED**

FLEXIBILITY · RELAXATION · MEDITATION

Activity Performed	Minutes
FLEXIBILITY · RELAXATION · MEDITATION TOTALS:	
COMMENTS:	

NUTRITIONAL INTAKE

Food Item	amt.	cal.	fat gms	protein gms	carbs gms	fiber gms
BREAKFAST:						
LUNCH:						
DINNER:						
SNACKS:						
INTAKE TOTALS:						

**VITAMINS &
SUPPLEMENTS**

Type: _____
Qty:

Type: _____
Qty:

Type: _____
Qty:

Type: _____
Qty:

WATER INTAKE:
OF 8OZ GLASSES

❑ ❑
❑ ❑
❑ ❑
❑ ❑
❑ ❑

COMMENTS · NOTES · PROGRESS

_____

_____

_____

_____

_____

DATE:_____ WEEK#:_____ DAY#:_____   WEIGHT:_____

ENERGY LEVELS: low ❑ med ❑ high ❑

Daily Workout Journal

Exercise
helps lower
cholesterol,
reduce blood
pressure,
and prevent
osteoporosis.

CARDIOVASCULAR EXERCISE   STRETCHING/WARMUP: yes ❑ no ❑

Time	Exercise Type	Minutes	Distance	Pace/ Setting	Cal. Burned
CARDIO EXERCISE TOTALS:					

COMMENTS:

STRENGTH TRAINING   TARGET AREA: upper body ❑ lower body ❑ abs ❑

Exercise Type	Muscle Group	SET 1 Reps/Wt.	SET 2 Reps/Wt.	SET 3 Reps/Wt.	SET 4 Reps/Wt.
STRENGTH TRAINING TOTALS:					

COMMENTS:

_____

_____

_____

_____

_____

_____

_____

_____

_____

_____

_____

OTHER · GROUP EXERCISE   STRETCHING/WARMUP: yes ❑ no ❑

Time	Exercise Type	Minutes	Cal. Burned
OTHER · GROUP EXERCISE TOTALS:			

COMMENTS:

DAILY GOAL(S) _____

_____

_____

**DAILY GOALS
ACHIEVED**

FLEXIBILITY · RELAXATION · MEDITATION

Activity Performed	Minutes
FLEXIBILITY · RELAXATION · MEDITATION TOTALS:	
COMMENTS:	

NUTRITIONAL INTAKE

Food Item	amt.	cal.	fat gms	protein gms	carbs gms	fiber gms
BREAKFAST:						
LUNCH:						
DINNER:						
SNACKS:						
INTAKE TOTALS:						

**VITAMINS &
SUPPLEMENTS**

Type: _____

Qty: _____

Type: _____

Qty: _____

Type: _____

Qty: _____

Type: _____

Qty: _____

WATER INTAKE:

OF 8OZ GLASSES

❏ ❏

❏ ❏

❏ ❏

❏ ❏

❏ ❏

COMMENTS · NOTES · PROGRESS

_____

_____

_____

_____

_____

DATE:_____ WEEK#:_____ DAY#:_____   WEIGHT:_____

ENERGY LEVELS: low ❑ med ❑ high ❑

Daily Workout Journal

CARDIOVASCULAR EXERCISE   STRETCHING/WARMUP: yes ❑ no ❑

Exercise
protects
against
arthritis,
heart disease,
breast
cancer and
numerous
other
diseases.

Time	Exercise Type	Minutes	Distance	Pace/ Setting	Cal. Burned
CARDIO EXERCISE TOTALS:					

COMMENTS:

STRENGTH TRAINING   TARGET AREA: upper body ❑ lower body ❑ abs ❑

Exercise Type	Muscle Group	SET 1 Reps/Wt.	SET 2 Reps/Wt.	SET 3 Reps/Wt.	SET 4 Reps/Wt.
STRENGTH TRAINING TOTALS:					

WORKOUT REMINDER:

_____

_____

_____

_____

COMMENTS:

OTHER · GROUP EXERCISE   STRETCHING/WARMUP: yes ❑ no ❑

_____

_____

_____

Time	Exercise Type	Minutes	Cal. Burned
OTHER · GROUP EXERCISE TOTALS:			

_____

COMMENTS:

DAILY GOALS
ACHIEVED

FLEXIBILITY · RELAXATION · MEDITATION

Activity Performed	Minutes
FLEXIBILITY · RELAXATION · MEDITATION TOTALS:	
COMMENTS:	

NUTRITIONAL INTAKE

Food Item	amt.	cal.	fat gms	protein gms	carbs gms	fiber gms
BREAKFAST:						
LUNCH:						
DINNER:						
SNACKS:						
INTAKE TOTALS:						

VITAMINS & SUPPLEMENTS

Type:

Qty:

Type:

Qty:

Type:

Qty:

Type:

Qty:

WATER INTAKE:
OF 8OZ GLASSES

❑ ❑

❑ ❑

❑ ❑

❑ ❑

❑ ❑

COMMENTS · NOTES · PROGRESS

ENERGY LEVELS: low ☐ med ☐ high ☐

Helpful Tips

Daily Workout Journal

CARDIOVASCULAR EXERCISE STRETCHING/WARMUP: yes ☐ no ☐

Increasing the body's lean muscle mass increases the body's ability to burn fat.

Time	Exercise Type	Minutes	Distance	Pace/Setting	Cal. Burned
CARDIO EXERCISE TOTALS:					

COMMENTS:

STRENGTH TRAINING TARGET AREA: upper body ☐ lower body ☐ abs ☐

Exercise Type	Muscle Group	SET 1 Reps/Wt.	SET 2 Reps/Wt.	SET 3 Reps/Wt.	SET 4 Reps/Wt.
STRENGTH TRAINING TOTALS:					

WORKOUT REMINDER:

_____

_____

_____

_____

_____

_____

COMMENTS:

OTHER · GROUP EXERCISE STRETCHING/WARMUP: yes ☐ no ☐

Time	Exercise Type	Minutes	Cal. Burned
OTHER · GROUP EXERCISE TOTALS:			

COMMENTS:

DAILY GOAL(S) _____

_____

_____

**DAILY GOALS
ACHIEVED**

FLEXIBILITY · RELAXATION · MEDITATION

Activity Performed	Minutes
FLEXIBILITY · RELAXATION · MEDITATION TOTALS:	
COMMENTS:	

NUTRITIONAL INTAKE

Food Item	amt.	cal.	fat gms	protein gms	carbs gms	fiber gms
BREAKFAST:						
LUNCH:						
DINNER:						
SNACKS:						
INTAKE TOTALS:						

VITAMINS & SUPPLEMENTS

Type: _____
Qty: _____

Type: _____
Qty: _____

Type: _____
Qty: _____

Type: _____
Qty: _____

WATER INTAKE:
OF 8OZ GLASSES

☐ ☐

☐ ☐

☐ ☐

☐ ☐

☐ ☐

COMMENTS · NOTES · PROGRESS

_____

_____

_____

_____

_____

DATE:_____ WEEK#:_____ DAY#:_____ WEIGHT:_____

ENERGY LEVELS: low ☐ med ☐ high ☐

Daily Workout Journal

Tests have
shown that
those who
maintain
a regular
exercise
routine
experience
more
consistent and
restful sleep.

CARDIOVASCULAR EXERCISE   STRETCHING/WARMUP: yes ☐ no ☐

Time	Exercise Type	Minutes	Distance	Pace/ Setting	Cal. Burned
CARDIO EXERCISE TOTALS:					

COMMENTS:

STRENGTH TRAINING   TARGET AREA: upper body ☐ lower body ☐ abs ☐

Exercise Type	Muscle Group	SET 1 Reps/Wt.	SET 2 Reps/Wt.	SET 3 Reps/Wt.	SET 4 Reps/Wt.
STRENGTH TRAINING TOTALS:					

COMMENTS:

OTHER · GROUP EXERCISE   STRETCHING/WARMUP: yes ☐ no ☐

Time	Exercise Type	Minutes	Cal. Burned
OTHER · GROUP EXERCISE TOTALS:			

COMMENTS:

**DAILY GOALS
ACHIEVED**

FLEXIBILITY · RELAXATION · MEDITATION

Activity Performed	Minutes
FLEXIBILITY · RELAXATION · MEDITATION TOTALS:	

COMMENTS:

NUTRITIONAL INTAKE

Food Item	amt.	cal.	fat gms	protein gms	carbs gms	fiber gms
BREAKFAST:						
LUNCH:						
DINNER:						
SNACKS:						
INTAKE TOTALS:						

VITAMINS & SUPPLEMENTS

Type:
Qty:

Type:
Qty:

Type:
Qty:

Type:
Qty:

WATER INTAKE:
OF 8oz GLASSES

☐ ☐
☐ ☐
☐ ☐
☐ ☐
☐ ☐

COMMENTS · NOTES · PROGRESS

DATE:_____ WEEK#:_____ DAY#:_____ WEIGHT:_____

ENERGY LEVELS: low ☐ med ☐ high ☐

Daily Workout Journal

Research
suggests
that exercise
increases the
body's ability
to produce
endorphins,
naturally
occurring
substances
that lower
anxiety, ease
depression,
and increase
self-esteem
and overall
happiness.

CARDIOVASCULAR EXERCISE   STRETCHING/WARMUP: yes ☐ no ☐

Time	Exercise Type	Minutes	Distance	Pace/ Setting	Cal. Burned
CARDIO EXERCISE TOTALS:					

COMMENTS:

STRENGTH TRAINING   TARGET AREA: upper body ☐ lower body ☐ abs ☐

Exercise Type	Muscle Group	SET 1 Reps/Wt.	SET 2 Reps/Wt.	SET 3 Reps/Wt.	SET 4 Reps/Wt.
STRENGTH TRAINING TOTALS:					

COMMENTS:

**WORKOUT
REMINDER:**

_____
_____
_____
_____
_____
_____
_____
_____
_____
_____
_____

OTHER · GROUP EXERCISE   STRETCHING/WARMUP: yes ☐ no ☐

Time	Exercise Type	Minutes	Cal. Burned
OTHER · GROUP EXERCISE TOTALS:			

COMMENTS:

DAILY GOAL(S)_____

_____

**DAILY GOALS
ACHIEVED**

FLEXIBILITY · RELAXATION · MEDITATION

Activity Performed	Minutes
FLEXIBILITY · RELAXATION · MEDITATION TOTALS:	
COMMENTS:	

NUTRITIONAL INTAKE

Food Item	amt.	cal.	fat gms	protein gms	carbs gms	fiber gms
BREAKFAST:						
LUNCH:						
DINNER:						
SNACKS:						
INTAKE TOTALS:						

**VITAMINS &
SUPPLEMENTS**

Type:_____
Qty:_____

Type:_____
Qty:_____

Type:_____
Qty:_____

Type:_____
Qty:_____

WATER INTAKE:
OF 8OZ GLASSES

❏ ❏

❏ ❏

❏ ❏

❏ ❏

❏ ❏

COMMENTS · NOTES · PROGRESS

_____

_____

_____

_____

_____

_____

DATE:_____ WEEK#:_____ DAY#:_____   WEIGHT:_____

Helpful Tips

Daily Workout Journal

A sedentary
lifestyle
increases
isolation,
while a
healthy,
active lifestyle
increases
opportunities
for social
interactions.

CARDIOVASCULAR EXERCISE   STRETCHING/WARMUP: yes ❑ no ❑

Time	Exercise Type	Minutes	Distance	Pace/ Setting	Cal. Burned
CARDIO EXERCISE TOTALS:					

COMMENTS:

STRENGTH TRAINING   TARGET AREA: upper body ❑ lower body ❑ abs ❑

Exercise Type	Muscle Group	SET 1 Reps/Wt.	SET 2 Reps/Wt.	SET 3 Reps/Wt.	SET 4 Reps/Wt.
STRENGTH TRAINING TOTALS:					

WORKOUT REMINDER:

_____

_____

_____

_____

_____

COMMENTS:

OTHER · GROUP EXERCISE   STRETCHING/WARMUP: yes ❑ no ❑

Time	Exercise Type	Minutes	Cal. Burned
OTHER·GROUP EXERCISE TOTALS:			

COMMENTS:

DAILY GOAL(S) _____

_____

_____

DAILY GOALS
ACHIEVED

FLEXIBILITY · RELAXATION · MEDITATION

Activity Performed	Minutes
FLEXIBILITY · RELAXATION · MEDITATION TOTALS:	
COMMENTS:	

NUTRITIONAL INTAKE

Food Item	amt.	cal.	fat gms	protein gms	carbs gms	fiber gms
BREAKFAST:						
LUNCH:						
DINNER:						
SNACKS:						
INTAKE TOTALS:						

VITAMINS & SUPPLEMENTS

Type: _____
Qty: _____

Type: _____
Qty: _____

Type: _____
Qty: _____

Type: _____
Qty: _____

WATER INTAKE:
OF 8OZ GLASSES

❑ ❑
❑ ❑
❑ ❑
❑ ❑
❑ ❑

COMMENTS · NOTES · PROGRESS

_____

_____

_____

_____

_____

ENERGY LEVELS: low ❑   med ❑   high ❑

Daily Workout Journal

CARDIOVASCULAR EXERCISE   STRETCHING/WARMUP: yes ❑   no ❑

Time	Exercise Type	Minutes	Distance	Pace/ Setting	Cal. Burned
CARDIO EXERCISE TOTALS:					

COMMENTS:

STRENGTH TRAINING   TARGET AREA: upper body ❑   lower body ❑   abs ❑

Exercise Type	Muscle Group	SET 1 Reps/Wt.	SET 2 Reps/Wt.	SET 3 Reps/Wt.	SET 4 Reps/Wt.
STRENGTH TRAINING TOTALS:					

COMMENTS:

OTHER · GROUP EXERCISE   STRETCHING/WARMUP: yes ❑   no ❑

Time	Exercise Type	Minutes	Cal. Burned
OTHER · GROUP EXERCISE TOTALS:			

COMMENTS:

DAILY GOAL(S) _____

_____

_____

DAILY GOALS
ACHIEVED

FLEXIBILITY · RELAXATION · MEDITATION

Activity Performed	Minutes
FLEXIBILITY · RELAXATION · MEDITATION TOTALS:	

COMMENTS:

NUTRITIONAL INTAKE

Food Item	amt.	cal.	fat gms	protein gms	carbs gms	fiber gms
BREAKFAST:						
LUNCH:						
DINNER:						
SNACKS:						
INTAKE TOTALS:						

VITAMINS & SUPPLEMENTS

Type: _____
Qty: _____

Type: _____
Qty: _____

Type: _____
Qty: _____

Type: _____
Qty: _____

WATER INTAKE:
OF 8OZ GLASSES

❏ ❏
❏ ❏
❏ ❏
❏ ❏
❏ ❏

COMMENTS · NOTES · PROGRESS

_____

_____

_____

_____

_____

DATE:_____ WEEK#:_____ DAY#:_____ WEIGHT:_____

ENERGY LEVELS: low ☐ med ☐ high ☐

Helpful Tips

Recent studies have shown that rapid fat loss from dieting without regular exercise may result in a significant loss in bone density. Maintaining a regular cardiovascular training program can eliminate this bone density loss and in some cases actually increase bone density.

WORKOUT REMINDER:

_____
_____
_____
_____
_____
_____
_____
_____
_____
_____
_____

CARDIOVASCULAR EXERCISE   STRETCHING/WARMUP: yes ☐ no ☐

Time	Exercise Type	Minutes	Distance	Pace/Setting	Cal. Burned
CARDIO EXERCISE TOTALS:					

COMMENTS:

STRENGTH TRAINING   TARGET AREA: upper body ☐ lower body ☐ abs ☐

Exercise Type	Muscle Group	SET 1 Reps/Wt.	SET 2 Reps/Wt.	SET 3 Reps/Wt.	SET 4 Reps/Wt.
STRENGTH TRAINING TOTALS:					

COMMENTS:

OTHER · GROUP EXERCISE   STRETCHING/WARMUP: yes ☐ no ☐

Time	Exercise Type	Minutes	Cal. Burned
OTHER · GROUP EXERCISE TOTALS:			

COMMENTS:

DAILY GOAL(S)_____

I DID IT!

DAILY GOALS
ACHIEVED

FLEXIBILITY · RELAXATION · MEDITATION

Activity Performed	Minutes
FLEXIBILITY · RELAXATION · MEDITATION TOTALS:	
COMMENTS:	

NUTRITIONAL INTAKE

Food Item	amt.	cal.	fat gms	protein gms	carbs gms	fiber gms
BREAKFAST:						
LUNCH:						
DINNER:						
SNACKS:						
INTAKE TOTALS:						

VITAMINS & SUPPLEMENTS

Type:_____
Qty:_____

Type:_____
Qty:_____

Type:_____
Qty:_____

Type:_____
Qty:_____

WATER INTAKE:

OF 8oz GLASSES

❑ ❑
❑ ❑
❑ ❑
❑ ❑
❑ ❑

COMMENTS · NOTES · PROGRESS

_____

_____

_____

_____

_____

DATE:_____ WEEK#:_____ DAY#:_____   WEIGHT:_____

ENERGY LEVELS: low ❑ med ❑ high ❑

Helpful Tips

Daily Workout Journal

Cardiovascular
training has
been shown
to decrease
the risk of
osteoporosis.

CARDIOVASCULAR EXERCISE STRETCHING/WARMUP: yes ❑ no ❑

Time	Exercise Type	Minutes	Distance	Pace/ Setting	Cal. Burned
CARDIO EXERCISE TOTALS:					

COMMENTS:

STRENGTH TRAINING TARGET AREA: upper body ❑ lower body ❑ abs ❑

Exercise Type	Muscle Group	SET 1 Reps/Wt.	SET 2 Reps/Wt.	SET 3 Reps/Wt.	SET 4 Reps/Wt.
STRENGTH TRAINING TOTALS:					

**WORKOUT
REMINDER:**

_____

_____

_____

_____

COMMENTS:

OTHER · GROUP EXERCISE STRETCHING/WARMUP: yes ❑ no ❑

Time	Exercise Type	Minutes	Cal. Burned
OTHER · GROUP EXERCISE TOTALS:			

COMMENTS:

DAILY GOAL(S) _____

_____

_____

DAILY GOALS ACHIEVED

FLEXIBILITY · RELAXATION · MEDITATION

Activity Performed	Minutes
FLEXIBILITY · RELAXATION · MEDITATION TOTALS:	

COMMENTS:

NUTRITIONAL INTAKE

Food Item	amt.	cal.	fat gms	protein gms	carbs gms	fiber gms
BREAKFAST:						
LUNCH:						
DINNER:						
SNACKS:						
INTAKE TOTALS:						

VITAMINS & SUPPLEMENTS

Type: _____

Qty: _____

Type: _____

Qty: _____

Type: _____

Qty: _____

Type: _____

Qty: _____

WATER INTAKE:

OF 8OZ GLASSES

☐ ☐
☐ ☐
☐ ☐
☐ ☐
☐ ☐

COMMENTS · NOTES · PROGRESS

_____

_____

_____

_____

_____

ENERGY LEVELS: low ☐ med ☐ high ☐

Helpful Tips

Daily Workout Journal

Strength training should work larger muscle groups before smaller muscles. If smaller muscles are worked first they will become fatigued and large muscles will not be able to work at their optimum capacity.

CARDIOVASCULAR EXERCISE   STRETCHING/WARMUP: yes ☐ no ☐

Time	Exercise Type	Minutes	Distance	Pace/ Setting	Cal. Burned
CARDIO EXERCISE TOTALS:					

COMMENTS:

STRENGTH TRAINING   TARGET AREA: upper body ☐ lower body ☐ abs ☐

Exercise Type	Muscle Group	SET 1 Reps/Wt.	SET 2 Reps/Wt.	SET 3 Reps/Wt.	SET 4 Reps/Wt.
STRENGTH TRAINING TOTALS:					

WORKOUT REMINDER:

_____

_____

_____

_____

_____

_____

_____

_____

_____

_____

COMMENTS:

OTHER · GROUP EXERCISE   STRETCHING/WARMUP: yes ☐ no ☐

Time	Exercise Type	Minutes	Cal. Burned
OTHER · GROUP EXERCISE TOTALS:			

COMMENTS:

DAILY GOAL(S) _____

_____

_____

DAILY GOALS
ACHIEVED

FLEXIBILITY · RELAXATION · MEDITATION

Activity Performed	Minutes
FLEXIBILITY · RELAXATION · MEDITATION TOTALS:	

COMMENTS:

NUTRITIONAL INTAKE

Food Item	amt.	cal.	fat gms	protein gms	carbs gms	fiber gms
BREAKFAST:						
LUNCH:						
DINNER:						
SNACKS:						
INTAKE TOTALS:						

VITAMINS & SUPPLEMENTS

Type: _____

Qty: _____

Type: _____

Qty: _____

Type: _____

Qty: _____

Type: _____

Qty: _____

WATER INTAKE:

OF 8OZ GLASSES

❏ ❏
❏ ❏
❏ ❏
❏ ❏
❏ ❏

COMMENTS · NOTES · PROGRESS

_____

_____

_____

_____

_____

ENERGY LEVELS: low ☐ med ☐ high ☐

Helpful Tips

Daily Workout Journal

CARDIOVASCULAR EXERCISE   STRETCHING/WARMUP: yes ☐ no ☐

Proper
flexibility
training
strengthens
tendons and
ligaments,
protects
muscle form,
and helps
prevent
muscles from
becoming
overly
exerted
(strained) or
contracted
(knotted).

Time	Exercise Type	Minutes	Distance	Pace/Setting	Cal. Burned
CARDIO EXERCISE TOTALS:					

COMMENTS:

STRENGTH TRAINING   TARGET AREA: upper body ☐ lower body ☐ abs ☐

Exercise Type	Muscle Group	SET 1 Reps/Wt.	SET 2 Reps/Wt.	SET 3 Reps/Wt.	SET 4 Reps/Wt.
STRENGTH TRAINING TOTALS:					

**WORKOUT
REMINDER:**

COMMENTS:

OTHER · GROUP EXERCISE   STRETCHING/WARMUP: yes ☐ no ☐

Time	Exercise Type	Minutes	Cal. Burned
OTHER · GROUP EXERCISE TOTALS:			

COMMENTS:

DAILY GOALS
ACHIEVED

FLEXIBILITY · RELAXATION · MEDITATION

Activity Performed	Minutes
FLEXIBILITY · RELAXATION · MEDITATION TOTALS:	

COMMENTS:

NUTRITIONAL INTAKE

Food Item	amt.	cal.	fat gms	protein gms	carbs gms	fiber gms
BREAKFAST:						
LUNCH:						
DINNER:						
SNACKS:						
INTAKE TOTALS:						

VITAMINS & SUPPLEMENTS

Type:
Qty:

Type:
Qty:

Type:
Qty:

Type:
Qty:

WATER INTAKE:

OF 8OZ GLASSES

❑ ❑
❑ ❑
❑ ❑
❑ ❑
❑ ❑

COMMENTS · NOTES · PROGRESS

DATE:_____ WEEK#:_____ DAY#:_____   WEIGHT:_____

Helpful Tips

Daily Workout Journal

Proper
stretching
reduces
tension
and helps
alleviate
stress.

CARDIOVASCULAR EXERCISE   STRETCHING/WARMUP: yes ☐ no ☐

Time	Exercise Type	Minutes	Distance	Pace/ Setting	Cal. Burned
CARDIO EXERCISE TOTALS:					

COMMENTS:

STRENGTH TRAINING   TARGET AREA: upper body ☐ lower body ☐ abs ☐

Exercise Type	Muscle Group	SET 1 Reps/Wt.	SET 2 Reps/Wt.	SET 3 Reps/Wt.	SET 4 Reps/Wt.
STRENGTH TRAINING TOTALS:					

**WORKOUT
REMINDER:**

_____

_____

_____

_____

COMMENTS:

OTHER · GROUP EXERCISE   STRETCHING/WARMUP: yes ☐ no ☐

_____

Time	Exercise Type	Minutes	Cal. Burned
OTHER · GROUP EXERCISE TOTALS:			

_____

COMMENTS:

DAILY GOAL(S) _____

_____

_____

DAILY GOALS
ACHIEVED

FLEXIBILITY · RELAXATION · MEDITATION

Activity Performed	Minutes
FLEXIBILITY · RELAXATION · MEDITATION TOTALS:	

COMMENTS:

NUTRITIONAL INTAKE

Food Item	amt.	cal.	fat gms	protein gms	carbs gms	fiber gms
BREAKFAST:						
LUNCH:						
DINNER:						
SNACKS:						
INTAKE TOTALS:						

VITAMINS & SUPPLEMENTS

Type: _____

Qty: _____

Type: _____

Qty: _____

Type: _____

Qty: _____

Type: _____

Qty: _____

WATER INTAKE:

OF 8OZ GLASSES

❏ ❏

❏ ❏

❏ ❏

❏ ❏

❏ ❏

COMMENTS · NOTES · PROGRESS

_____

_____

_____

_____

_____

DATE:_____ WEEK#:_____ DAY#:_____ WEIGHT:_____

ENERGY LEVELS: low ☐ med ☐ high ☐

Daily Workout Journal

Sudden
jerking or
bouncing
during
stretching
can increase
the chance of
injury. All
stretching
motions
should be
fluid and
without
sudden
acceleration
or
deceleration.

CARDIOVASCULAR EXERCISE   STRETCHING/WARMUP: yes ☐ no ☐

Time	Exercise Type	Minutes	Distance	Pace/ Setting	Cal. Burned
CARDIO EXERCISE TOTALS:					

COMMENTS:

STRENGTH TRAINING   TARGET AREA: upper body ☐ lower body ☐ abs ☐

Exercise Type	Muscle Group	SET 1 Reps/Wt.	SET 2 Reps/Wt.	SET 3 Reps/Wt.	SET 4 Reps/Wt.
STRENGTH TRAINING TOTALS:					

COMMENTS:

OTHER · GROUP EXERCISE   STRETCHING/WARMUP: yes ☐ no ☐

Time	Exercise Type	Minutes	Cal. Burned
OTHER · GROUP EXERCISE TOTALS:			

COMMENTS:

DAILY GOAL(S) _____

_____

_____

**DAILY GOALS
ACHIEVED**

FLEXIBILITY · RELAXATION · MEDITATION

Activity Performed	Minutes
FLEXIBILITY · RELAXATION · MEDITATION TOTALS:	
COMMENTS:	

NUTRITIONAL INTAKE

Food Item	amt.	cal.	fat gms	protein gms	carbs gms	fiber gms
BREAKFAST:						
LUNCH:						
DINNER:						
SNACKS:						
INTAKE TOTALS:						

VITAMINS & SUPPLEMENTS

Type: _____
Qty: _____

Type: _____
Qty: _____

Type: _____
Qty: _____

Type: _____
Qty: _____

WATER INTAKE:
OF 8OZ GLASSES

❏ ❏
❏ ❏
❏ ❏
❏ ❏
❏ ❏

COMMENTS · NOTES · PROGRESS

_____

_____

_____

_____

_____

DATE:_____ WEEK#:_____ DAY#:_____   WEIGHT:_____

Helpful Tips

Daily Workout Journal

CARDIOVASCULAR EXERCISE   STRETCHING/WARMUP: yes ☐ no ☐

Stretches
should
exceed
normal
comfort
levels, but
not to the
point of
pain. The
body should
experience
only mild
discomfort
while
stretching.

Time	Exercise Type	Minutes	Distance	Pace/ Setting	Cal. Burned
CARDIO EXERCISE TOTALS:					

COMMENTS:

STRENGTH TRAINING   TARGET AREA: upper body ☐ lower body ☐ abs ☐

Exercise Type	Muscle Group	SET 1 Reps/Wt.	SET 2 Reps/Wt.	SET 3 Reps/Wt.	SET 4 Reps/Wt.
STRENGTH TRAINING TOTALS:					

**WORKOUT
REMINDER:**

_____

_____

_____

_____

_____

_____

_____

COMMENTS:

OTHER · GROUP EXERCISE   STRETCHING/WARMUP: yes ☐ no ☐

Time	Exercise Type	Minutes	Cal. Burned
OTHER · GROUP EXERCISE TOTALS:			

COMMENTS:

DAILY GOAL(S)_____

_____

_____

I DID IT!

**DAILY GOALS
ACHIEVED**

FLEXIBILITY · RELAXATION · MEDITATION

Activity Performed	Minutes
FLEXIBILITY · RELAXATION · MEDITATION TOTALS:	

COMMENTS:

NUTRITIONAL INTAKE

Food Item	amt.	cal.	fat gms	protein gms	carbs gms	fiber gms
BREAKFAST:						
LUNCH:						
DINNER:						
SNACKS:						
INTAKE TOTALS:						

**VITAMINS &
SUPPLEMENTS**

Type:_____

Qty:_____

Type:_____

Qty:_____

Type:_____

Qty:_____

Type:_____

Qty:_____

WATER INTAKE:

OF 8OZ GLASSES

❑ ❑

❑ ❑

❑ ❑

❑ ❑

❑ ❑

COMMENTS · NOTES · PROGRESS

_____

_____

_____

_____

_____

DATE:_____ WEEK#:_____ DAY#:_____   WEIGHT:_____

ENERGY LEVELS: low ☐ med ☐ high ☐

Helpful Tips

Daily Workout Journal

Restaurant entrée portions are usually twice as large as what your body requires. When eating a large meal at a restaurant, simply divide the entrée in half. Take half home and have it for another meal.

CARDIOVASCULAR EXERCISE   STRETCHING/WARMUP: yes ☐ no ☐

Time	Exercise Type	Minutes	Distance	Pace/Setting	Cal. Burned
CARDIO EXERCISE TOTALS:					

COMMENTS:

STRENGTH TRAINING   TARGET AREA: upper body ☐ lower body ☐ abs ☐

Exercise Type	Muscle Group	SET 1 Reps/Wt.	SET 2 Reps/Wt.	SET 3 Reps/Wt.	SET 4 Reps/Wt.
STRENGTH TRAINING TOTALS:					

COMMENTS:

WORKOUT REMINDER:

_____

_____

_____

_____

_____

_____

_____

OTHER · GROUP EXERCISE   STRETCHING/WARMUP: yes ☐ no ☐

Time	Exercise Type	Minutes	Cal. Burned
OTHER · GROUP EXERCISE TOTALS:			

COMMENTS:

DAILY GOAL(S) _____

_____

_____

DAILY GOALS
ACHIEVED

FLEXIBILITY · RELAXATION · MEDITATION

Activity Performed	Minutes
FLEXIBILITY · RELAXATION · MEDITATION TOTALS:	
COMMENTS:	

NUTRITIONAL INTAKE

Food Item	amt.	cal.	fat gms	protein gms	carbs gms	fiber gms
BREAKFAST:						
LUNCH:						
DINNER:						
SNACKS:						
INTAKE TOTALS:						

VITAMINS & SUPPLEMENTS

Type: _____

Qty: _____

Type: _____

Qty: _____

Type: _____

Qty: _____

Type: _____

Qty: _____

WATER INTAKE:

OF 8OZ GLASSES

❏ ❏

❏ ❏

❏ ❏

❏ ❏

❏ ❏

COMMENTS · NOTES · PROGRESS

_____

_____

_____

_____

_____

DATE:_____ WEEK#:_____ DAY#:_____ WEIGHT:_____

ENERGY LEVELS: low ☐ med ☐ high ☐

Daily Workout Journal

CARDIOVASCULAR EXERCISE STRETCHING/WARMUP: yes ☐ no ☐

In order to
lose one
pound, you
must burn
3500 more
calories than
you take in.
Conversely,
those looking
to gain
weight must
take in 3500
more calories
than they
burn.

Time	Exercise Type	Minutes	Distance	Pace/ Setting	Cal. Burned
CARDIO EXERCISE TOTALS:					

COMMENTS:

STRENGTH TRAINING TARGET AREA: upper body ☐ lower body ☐ abs ☐

Exercise Type	Muscle Group	SET 1 Reps/Wt.	SET 2 Reps/Wt.	SET 3 Reps/Wt.	SET 4 Reps/Wt.
STRENGTH TRAINING TOTALS:					

WORKOUT REMINDER:

_____

_____

_____

_____

_____

COMMENTS:

OTHER · GROUP EXERCISE STRETCHING/WARMUP: yes ☐ no ☐

_____

_____

_____

_____

_____

Time	Exercise Type	Minutes	Cal. Burned
OTHER · GROUP EXERCISE TOTALS:			

COMMENTS:

DAILY GOAL(S) _____

_____

I DID IT!

DAILY GOALS ACHIEVED

FLEXIBILITY · RELAXATION · MEDITATION

Activity Performed	Minutes
FLEXIBILITY · RELAXATION · MEDITATION TOTALS:	

COMMENTS:

NUTRITIONAL INTAKE

Food Item	amt.	cal.	fat gms	protein gms	carbs gms	fiber gms
BREAKFAST:						
LUNCH:						
DINNER:						
SNACKS:						
INTAKE TOTALS:						

VITAMINS & SUPPLEMENTS

Type: _____

Qty: _____

Type: _____

Qty: _____

Type: _____

Qty: _____

Type: _____

Qty: _____

WATER INTAKE:

OF 8OZ GLASSES

❑ ❑

❑ ❑

❑ ❑

❑ ❑

❑ ❑

COMMENTS · NOTES · PROGRESS

_____

_____

_____

_____

_____

DATE:_____ WEEK#:_____ DAY#:_____   WEIGHT:_____

ENERGY LEVELS: low ☐   med ☐   high ☐

Daily Workout Journal

Your body's
Basal
Metabolic
Rate (BMR)
is the amount
of energy
used by the
body to
maintain
normal body
function
while at rest.
This typically
represents
about 70
percent of
all calories
consumed.

CARDIOVASCULAR EXERCISE   STRETCHING/WARMUP: yes ☐   no ☐

Time	Exercise Type	Minutes	Distance	Pace/ Setting	Cal. Burned
CARDIO EXERCISE TOTALS:					

COMMENTS:

STRENGTH TRAINING   TARGET AREA: upper body ☐   lower body ☐   abs ☐

Exercise Type	Muscle Group	SET 1 Reps/Wt.	SET 2 Reps/Wt.	SET 3 Reps/Wt.	SET 4 Reps/Wt.
STRENGTH TRAINING TOTALS:					

COMMENTS:

OTHER·GROUP EXERCISE   STRETCHING/WARMUP: yes ☐   no ☐

Time	Exercise Type	Minutes	Cal. Burned
OTHER·GROUP EXERCISE TOTALS:			

COMMENTS:

DAILY GOAL(S) _____

_____

_____

**DAILY GOALS
ACHIEVED**

FLEXIBILITY · RELAXATION · MEDITATION

Activity Performed	Minutes
FLEXIBILITY · RELAXATION · MEDITATION TOTALS:	
COMMENTS:	

NUTRITIONAL INTAKE

Food Item	amt.	cal.	fat gms	protein gms	carbs gms	fiber gms
BREAKFAST:						
LUNCH:						
DINNER:						
SNACKS:						
INTAKE TOTALS:						

**VITAMINS &
SUPPLEMENTS**

Type: _____

Qty: _____

Type: _____

Qty: _____

Type: _____

Qty: _____

Type: _____

Qty: _____

Type: _____

Qty: _____

WATER INTAKE:

OF 8oz GLASSES

❏ ❏

❏ ❏

❏ ❏

❏ ❏

❏ ❏

COMMENTS · NOTES · PROGRESS

_____

_____

_____

_____

_____

_____

DATE:_____ WEEK#:_____ DAY#:_____   WEIGHT:_____

Helpful Tips

Daily Workout Journal

Eating more
frequently
throughout
the day
causes your
body's
digestive
system to
stay active
for longer
periods,
therefore
burning more
calories than
if you eat
two or three
larger meals.

CARDIOVASCULAR EXERCISE STRETCHING/WARMUP: yes ☐ no ☐

Time	Exercise Type	Minutes	Distance	Pace/Setting	Cal. Burned
CARDIO EXERCISE TOTALS:					

COMMENTS:

STRENGTH TRAINING TARGET AREA: upper body ☐ lower body ☐ abs ☐

Exercise Type	Muscle Group	SET 1 Reps/Wt.	SET 2 Reps/Wt.	SET 3 Reps/Wt.	SET 4 Reps/Wt.
STRENGTH TRAINING TOTALS:					

**WORKOUT
REMINDER:**

_____

_____

_____

_____

_____

COMMENTS:

_____

_____

OTHER·GROUP EXERCISE STRETCHING/WARMUP: yes ☐ no ☐

_____

Time	Exercise Type	Minutes	Cal. Burned
OTHER·GROUP EXERCISE TOTALS:			

_____

COMMENTS:

DAILY GOAL(S) _____

_____

_____

**DAILY GOALS
ACHIEVED**

FLEXIBILITY · RELAXATION · MEDITATION

Activity Performed	Minutes
FLEXIBILITY · RELAXATION · MEDITATION TOTALS:	
COMMENTS:	

NUTRITIONAL INTAKE

Food Item	amt.	cal.	fat gms	protein gms	carbs gms	fiber gms
BREAKFAST:						
LUNCH:						
DINNER:						
SNACKS:						
INTAKE TOTALS:						

**VITAMINS &
SUPPLEMENTS**

Type: _____

Qty: _____

Type: _____

Qty: _____

Type: _____

Qty: _____

Type: _____

Qty: _____

WATER INTAKE:

OF 8OZ GLASSES

❏ ❏

❏ ❏

❏ ❏

❏ ❏

❏ ❏

COMMENTS · NOTES · PROGRESS

_____

_____

_____

_____

_____

DATE:_____ WEEK#:_____ DAY#:_____   WEIGHT:_____

ENERGY LEVELS: low ❑   med ❑   high ❑

Daily Workout Journal

CARDIOVASCULAR EXERCISE   STRETCHING/WARMUP: yes ❑ no ❑

Time	Exercise Type	Minutes	Distance	Pace/ Setting	Cal. Burned
CARDIO EXERCISE TOTALS:					

COMMENTS:

STRENGTH TRAINING   TARGET AREA: upper body ❑ lower body ❑ abs ❑

Exercise Type	Muscle Group	SET 1 Reps/Wt.	SET 2 Reps/Wt.	SET 3 Reps/Wt.	SET 4 Reps/Wt.
STRENGTH TRAINING TOTALS:					

WORKOUT REMINDER:

_____

_____

_____

_____

_____

_____

_____

_____

_____

COMMENTS:

OTHER · GROUP EXERCISE   STRETCHING/WARMUP: yes ❑ no ❑

Time	Exercise Type	Minutes	Cal. Burned
OTHER · GROUP EXERCISE TOTALS:			

COMMENTS:

DAILY GOAL(S) _____

_____

_____

DAILY GOALS ACHIEVED

FLEXIBILITY · RELAXATION · MEDITATION

Activity Performed	Minutes
FLEXIBILITY · RELAXATION · MEDITATION TOTALS:	
COMMENTS:	

NUTRITIONAL INTAKE

Food Item	amt.	cal.	fat gms	protein gms	carbs gms	fiber gms
BREAKFAST:						
LUNCH:						
DINNER:						
SNACKS:						
INTAKE TOTALS:						

VITAMINS & SUPPLEMENTS

Type: _____

Qty: _____

Type: _____

Qty: _____

Type: _____

Qty: _____

Type: _____

Qty: _____

WATER INTAKE:

OF 8OZ GLASSES

❏ ❏
❏ ❏
❏ ❏
❏ ❏
❏ ❏

COMMENTS · NOTES · PROGRESS

_____

_____

_____

_____

_____

DATE:_____ WEEK#:_____ DAY#:_____ WEIGHT:_____

Helpful Tips

Daily Workout Journal

Experts agree that taking a daily multivitamin is an excellent way to maintain proper nutrition or supplement a vitamin-deficient diet.

CARDIOVASCULAR EXERCISE   STRETCHING/WARMUP: yes ❏ no ❏

Time	Exercise Type	Minutes	Distance	Pace/ Setting	Cal. Burned
CARDIO EXERCISE TOTALS:					

COMMENTS:

STRENGTH TRAINING   TARGET AREA: upper body ❏ lower body ❏ abs ❏

Exercise Type	Muscle Group	SET 1 Reps/Wt.	SET 2 Reps/Wt.	SET 3 Reps/Wt.	SET 4 Reps/Wt.
STRENGTH TRAINING TOTALS:					

WORKOUT REMINDER:

_____

_____

_____

_____

_____

_____

_____

_____

_____

_____

COMMENTS:

OTHER · GROUP EXERCISE   STRETCHING/WARMUP: yes ❏ no ❏

Time	Exercise Type	Minutes	Cal. Burned
OTHER · GROUP EXERCISE TOTALS:			

COMMENTS:

DAILY GOAL(S) _____

_____

_____

DAILY GOALS ACHIEVED

FLEXIBILITY · RELAXATION · MEDITATION

Activity Performed	Minutes
FLEXIBILITY · RELAXATION · MEDITATION TOTALS:	
COMMENTS:	

NUTRITIONAL INTAKE

Food Item	amt.	cal.	fat gms	protein gms	carbs gms	fiber gms
BREAKFAST:						
LUNCH:						
DINNER:	.					
SNACKS:						
INTAKE TOTALS:						

VITAMINS & SUPPLEMENTS

Type: _____

Qty: _____

Type: _____

Qty: _____

Type: _____

Qty: _____

Type: _____

Qty: _____

WATER INTAKE:

OF 8OZ GLASSES

☐ ☐

☐ ☐

☐ ☐

☐ ☐

☐ ☐

COMMENTS · NOTES · PROGRESS

_____

_____

_____

_____

_____

_____

DATE:_____ WEEK#:_____ DAY#:_____   WEIGHT:_____

ENERGY LEVELS: low ☐ med ☐ high ☐

Daily Workout Journal

Stay
hydrated.
Water is
crucial to
all of the
body's major
functions
down to the
cellular level.

CARDIOVASCULAR EXERCISE   STRETCHING/WARMUP: yes ☐ no ☐

Time	Exercise Type	Minutes	Distance	Pace/ Setting	Cal. Burned
CARDIO EXERCISE TOTALS:					

COMMENTS:

STRENGTH TRAINING   TARGET AREA: upper body ☐ lower body ☐ abs ☐

Exercise Type	Muscle Group	SET 1 Reps/Wt.	SET 2 Reps/Wt.	SET 3 Reps/Wt.	SET 4 Reps/Wt.
STRENGTH TRAINING TOTALS:					

COMMENTS:

OTHER · GROUP EXERCISE   STRETCHING/WARMUP: yes ☐ no ☐

Time	Exercise Type	Minutes	Cal. Burned
OTHER · GROUP EXERCISE TOTALS:			

COMMENTS:

DAILY GOAL(S) _____

_____

DAILY GOALS
ACHIEVED

FLEXIBILITY · RELAXATION · MEDITATION

Activity Performed	Minutes
FLEXIBILITY · RELAXATION · MEDITATION TOTALS:	

COMMENTS:

NUTRITIONAL INTAKE

Food Item	amt.	cal.	fat gms	protein gms	carbs gms	fiber gms
BREAKFAST:						
LUNCH:						
DINNER:						
SNACKS:						
INTAKE TOTALS:						

VITAMINS & SUPPLEMENTS

Type: _____
Qty: _____

Type: _____
Qty: _____

Type: _____
Qty: _____

Type: _____
Qty: _____

WATER INTAKE:

OF 8OZ GLASSES

❑ ❑
❑ ❑
❑ ❑
❑ ❑
❑ ❑

COMMENTS · NOTES · PROGRESS

_____

_____

_____

_____

_____

DATE:_____ WEEK#:_____ DAY#:_____ WEIGHT:_____

Daily Workout Journal

CARDIOVASCULAR EXERCISE   STRETCHING/WARMUP: yes ☐ no ☐

Time	Exercise Type	Minutes	Distance	Pace/ Setting	Cal. Burned
CARDIO EXERCISE TOTALS:					

COMMENTS:

STRENGTH TRAINING   TARGET AREA: upper body ☐ lower body ☐ abs ☐

Exercise Type	Muscle Group	SET 1 Reps/Wt.	SET 2 Reps/Wt.	SET 3 Reps/Wt.	SET 4 Reps/Wt.
STRENGTH TRAINING TOTALS:					

WORKOUT REMINDER:

_____

_____

_____

_____

_____

_____

COMMENTS:

OTHER · GROUP EXERCISE   STRETCHING/WARMUP: yes ☐ no ☐

Time	Exercise Type	Minutes	Cal. Burned
OTHER · GROUP EXERCISE TOTALS:			

COMMENTS:

DAILY GOAL(S) _____

I DID IT!

DAILY GOALS
ACHIEVED

FLEXIBILITY · RELAXATION · MEDITATION

Activity Performed	Minutes
FLEXIBILITY · RELAXATION · MEDITATION TOTALS:	
COMMENTS:	

NUTRITIONAL INTAKE

Food Item	amt.	cal.	fat gms	protein gms	carbs gms	fiber gms
BREAKFAST:						
LUNCH:						
DINNER:						
SNACKS:						
INTAKE TOTALS:						

VITAMINS & SUPPLEMENTS

Type: _____
Qty: _____

Type: _____
Qty: _____

Type: _____
Qty: _____

Type: _____
Qty: _____

WATER INTAKE:
OF 8OZ GLASSES

❏ ❏
❏ ❏
❏ ❏
❏ ❏
❏ ❏

COMMENTS · NOTES · PROGRESS

_____

_____

_____

_____

_____

ENERGY LEVELS: low ❏ med ❏ high ❏

Helpful Tips

Daily Workout Journal

Experts say that men should drink around 120 ounces of water every day; women should drink around 90 ounces every day.

CARDIOVASCULAR EXERCISE STRETCHING/WARMUP: yes ❏ no ❏

Time	Exercise Type	Minutes	Distance	Pace/ Setting	Cal. Burned
CARDIO EXERCISE TOTALS:					

COMMENTS:

STRENGTH TRAINING TARGET AREA: upper body ❏ lower body ❏ abs ❏

Exercise Type	Muscle Group	SET 1 Reps/Wt.	SET 2 Reps/Wt.	SET 3 Reps/Wt.	SET 4 Reps/Wt.
STRENGTH TRAINING TOTALS:					

WORKOUT REMINDER:

_____

_____

_____

_____

_____

_____

_____

_____

_____

COMMENTS:

OTHER · GROUP EXERCISE STRETCHING/WARMUP: yes ❏ no ❏

Time	Exercise Type	Minutes	Cal. Burned
OTHER · GROUP EXERCISE TOTALS:			

COMMENTS:

DAILY GOAL(S) _____

_____

_____

DAILY GOALS
ACHIEVED

FLEXIBILITY · RELAXATION · MEDITATION

Activity Performed	Minutes
FLEXIBILITY · RELAXATION · MEDITATION TOTALS:	
COMMENTS:	

NUTRITIONAL INTAKE

Food Item	amt.	cal.	fat gms	protein gms	carbs gms	fiber gms
BREAKFAST:						
LUNCH:						
DINNER:						
SNACKS:						
INTAKE TOTALS:						

VITAMINS & SUPPLEMENTS

Type: _____
Qty: _____

Type: _____
Qty: _____

Type: _____
Qty: _____

Type: _____
Qty: _____

WATER INTAKE:
OF 8OZ GLASSES

❏ ❏
❏ ❏
❏ ❏
❏ ❏
❏ ❏

COMMENTS · NOTES · PROGRESS

_____

_____

_____

_____

_____

_____

DATE:_____ WEEK#:_____ DAY#:_____   WEIGHT:_____

ENERGY LEVELS: low ☐ med ☐ high ☐

Daily Workout Journal

CARDIOVASCULAR EXERCISE   STRETCHING/WARMUP: yes ☐ no ☐

Remember
to increase
your water
consumption
when
conditions
(e.g., hot
weather, high
altitude, low
humidity,
or increased
physical
activity) cause
you to lose
water more
rapidly than
normal.

Time	Exercise Type	Minutes	Distance	Pace/Setting	Cal. Burned
CARDIO EXERCISE TOTALS:					

COMMENTS:

STRENGTH TRAINING   TARGET AREA: upper body ☐ lower body ☐ abs ☐

Exercise Type	Muscle Group	SET 1 Reps/Wt.	SET 2 Reps/Wt.	SET 3 Reps/Wt.	SET 4 Reps/Wt.
STRENGTH TRAINING TOTALS:					

COMMENTS:

OTHER · GROUP EXERCISE   STRETCHING/WARMUP: yes ☐ no ☐

Time	Exercise Type	Minutes	Cal. Burned
OTHER · GROUP EXERCISE TOTALS:			

COMMENTS:

**DAILY GOALS
ACHIEVED**

FLEXIBILITY · RELAXATION · MEDITATION

Activity Performed	Minutes
FLEXIBILITY · RELAXATION · MEDITATION TOTALS:	
COMMENTS:	

NUTRITIONAL INTAKE

Food Item	amt.	cal.	fat gms	protein gms	carbs gms	fiber gms
BREAKFAST:						
LUNCH:						
DINNER:						
SNACKS:						
INTAKE TOTALS:						

VITAMINS & SUPPLEMENTS

Type: _____
Qty: _____

Type: _____
Qty: _____

Type: _____
Qty: _____

Type: _____
Qty: _____

WATER INTAKE:

OF 8OZ GLASSES

❑ ❑
❑ ❑
❑ ❑
❑ ❑
❑ ❑

COMMENTS · NOTES · PROGRESS

_____
_____
_____
_____
_____

DATE:_____ WEEK#:_____ DAY#:_____ WEIGHT:_____

ENERGY LEVELS: low ☐ med ☐ high ☐

Helpful Tips

Daily Workout Journal

Caffeinated drinks like coffee, tea and many soft drinks are actually diuretics, meaning that they increase fluid loss. In order to maintain proper hydration, limit the amount of caffeinated beverages and drink more water to compensate.

CARDIOVASCULAR EXERCISE   STRETCHING/WARMUP: yes ☐ no ☐

Time	Exercise Type	Minutes	Distance	Pace/ Setting	Cal. Burned
CARDIO EXERCISE TOTALS:					

COMMENTS:

STRENGTH TRAINING   TARGET AREA: upper body ☐ lower body ☐ abs ☐

Exercise Type	Muscle Group	SET 1 Reps/Wt.	SET 2 Reps/Wt.	SET 3 Reps/Wt.	SET 4 Reps/Wt.
STRENGTH TRAINING TOTALS:					

COMMENTS:

WORKOUT REMINDER:

_____

_____

_____

_____

_____

_____

_____

_____

_____

_____

_____

OTHER · GROUP EXERCISE   STRETCHING/WARMUP: yes ☐ no ☐

Time	Exercise Type	Minutes	Cal. Burned
OTHER · GROUP EXERCISE TOTALS:			

COMMENTS:

DAILY GOAL(S) _____

_____

**DAILY GOALS
ACHIEVED**

FLEXIBILITY · RELAXATION · MEDITATION

Activity Performed	Minutes
FLEXIBILITY · RELAXATION · MEDITATION TOTALS:	
COMMENTS:	

NUTRITIONAL INTAKE

Food Item	amt.	cal.	fat gms	protein gms	carbs gms	fiber gms
BREAKFAST:						
LUNCH:						
DINNER:						
SNACKS:						
INTAKE TOTALS:						

**VITAMINS &
SUPPLEMENTS**

Type: _____

Qty: _____

Type: _____

Qty: _____

Type: _____

Qty: _____

Type: _____

Qty: _____

WATER INTAKE:

OF 8OZ GLASSES

❏ ❏

❏ ❏

❏ ❏

❏ ❏

❏ ❏

COMMENTS · NOTES · PROGRESS

_____

_____

_____

_____

_____

ENERGY LEVELS: low ☐ med ☐ high ☐

Helpful Tips

Daily Workout Journal

You should drink 4-8 ounces of water every fifteen minutes while working out. During vigorous cardiovascular training, or if exercising in hot temperatures, increase your water consumption in order to replace water lost from sweating.

CARDIOVASCULAR EXERCISE   STRETCHING/WARMUP: yes ☐ no ☐

Time	Exercise Type	Minutes	Distance	Pace/ Setting	Cal. Burned
CARDIO EXERCISE TOTALS:					

COMMENTS:

STRENGTH TRAINING   TARGET AREA: upper body ☐ lower body ☐ abs ☐

Exercise Type	Muscle Group	SET 1 Reps/Wt.	SET 2 Reps/Wt.	SET 3 Reps/Wt.	SET 4 Reps/Wt.
STRENGTH TRAINING TOTALS:					

WORKOUT REMINDER:

_____

_____

_____

_____

_____

COMMENTS:

OTHER · GROUP EXERCISE   STRETCHING/WARMUP: yes ☐ no ☐

_____

_____

Time	Exercise Type	Minutes	Cal. Burned
OTHER · GROUP EXERCISE TOTALS:			

_____

COMMENTS:

DAILY GOAL(S) _____

_____

I DID IT!

DAILY GOALS
ACHIEVED

FLEXIBILITY · RELAXATION · MEDITATION

Activity Performed	Minutes
FLEXIBILITY · RELAXATION · MEDITATION TOTALS:	

COMMENTS:

NUTRITIONAL INTAKE

Food Item	amt.	cal.	fat gms	protein gms	carbs gms	fiber gms
BREAKFAST:						
LUNCH:						
DINNER:						
SNACKS:						
INTAKE TOTALS:						

VITAMINS & SUPPLEMENTS

Type: _____
Qty: _____

Type: _____
Qty: _____

Type: _____
Qty: _____

Type: _____
Qty: _____

WATER INTAKE:

OF 8OZ GLASSES

☐ ☐
☐ ☐
☐ ☐
☐ ☐
☐ ☐

COMMENTS · NOTES · PROGRESS

_____

_____

_____

_____

_____

_____

ENERGY LEVELS: low ❑ med ❑ high ❑

Daily Workout Journal

CARDIOVASCULAR EXERCISE STRETCHING/WARMUP: yes ❑ no ❑

Time	Exercise Type	Minutes	Distance	Pace/ Setting	Cal. Burned
CARDIO EXERCISE TOTALS:					

COMMENTS:

STRENGTH TRAINING TARGET AREA: upper body ❑ lower body ❑ abs ❑

Exercise Type	Muscle Group	SET 1 Reps/Wt.	SET 2 Reps/Wt.	SET 3 Reps/Wt.	SET 4 Reps/Wt.
STRENGTH TRAINING TOTALS:					

COMMENTS:

OTHER · GROUP EXERCISE STRETCHING/WARMUP: yes ❑ no ❑

Time	Exercise Type	Minutes	Cal. Burned
OTHER·GROUP EXERCISE TOTALS:			

COMMENTS:

I DID IT!

DAILY GOALS
ACHIEVED

FLEXIBILITY · RELAXATION · MEDITATION

Activity Performed	Minutes
FLEXIBILITY · RELAXATION · MEDITATION TOTALS:	

COMMENTS:

NUTRITIONAL INTAKE

Food Item	amt.	cal.	fat gms	protein gms	carbs gms	fiber gms
BREAKFAST:						
LUNCH:						
DINNER:						
SNACKS:						
INTAKE TOTALS:						

VITAMINS & SUPPLEMENTS

Type: _____
Qty: _____

Type: _____
Qty: _____

Type: _____
Qty: _____

Type: _____
Qty: _____

WATER INTAKE:

OF 8OZ GLASSES

❏ ❏

❏ ❏

❏ ❏

❏ ❏

❏ ❏

COMMENTS · NOTES · PROGRESS

_____
_____
_____
_____
_____
_____

DATE:_____ WEEK#:_____ DAY#:_____ WEIGHT:_____

Helpful Tips

Daily Workout Journal

Drinking 8
– 16 ounces
of water
within thirty
minutes of
completing
your exercise
routine helps
prevent
muscle
soreness.

CARDIOVASCULAR EXERCISE   STRETCHING/WARMUP: yes ☐ no ☐

Time	Exercise Type	Minutes	Distance	Pace/ Setting	Cal. Burned
CARDIO EXERCISE TOTALS:					

COMMENTS:

STRENGTH TRAINING   TARGET AREA: upper body ☐ lower body ☐ abs ☐

Exercise Type	Muscle Group	SET 1 Reps/Wt.	SET 2 Reps/Wt.	SET 3 Reps/Wt.	SET 4 Reps/Wt.
STRENGTH TRAINING TOTALS:					

WORKOUT REMINDER:

_____

_____

_____

_____

_____

COMMENTS:

OTHER · GROUP EXERCISE   STRETCHING/WARMUP: yes ☐ no ☐

Time	Exercise Type	Minutes	Cal. Burned
OTHER · GROUP EXERCISE TOTALS:			

_____

_____

_____

_____

COMMENTS:

DAILY GOAL(S) _____

_____

_____

DAILY GOALS
ACHIEVED

FLEXIBILITY · RELAXATION · MEDITATION

Activity Performed	Minutes
FLEXIBILITY · RELAXATION · MEDITATION TOTALS:	
COMMENTS:	

NUTRITIONAL INTAKE

Food Item	amt.	cal.	fat gms	protein gms	carbs gms	fiber gms
BREAKFAST:						
LUNCH:						
DINNER:						
SNACKS:						
INTAKE TOTALS:						

VITAMINS & SUPPLEMENTS

Type: _____

Qty: _____

Type: _____

Qty: _____

Type: _____

Qty: _____

Type: _____

Qty: _____

WATER INTAKE:

OF 8OZ GLASSES

☐ ☐

☐ ☐

☐ ☐

☐ ☐

☐ ☐

COMMENTS · NOTES · PROGRESS

_____

_____

_____

_____

_____

DATE:_____ WEEK#:_____ DAY#:_____ WEIGHT:_____

ENERGY LEVELS: low ❑ med ❑ high ❑

Daily Workout Journal

CARDIOVASCULAR EXERCISE   STRETCHING/WARMUP: yes ❑ no ❑

Time	Exercise Type	Minutes	Distance	Pace/Setting	Cal. Burned
CARDIO EXERCISE TOTALS:					

COMMENTS:

STRENGTH TRAINING   TARGET AREA: upper body ❑ lower body ❑ abs ❑

Exercise Type	Muscle Group	SET 1 Reps/Wt.	SET 2 Reps/Wt.	SET 3 Reps/Wt.	SET 4 Reps/Wt.
STRENGTH TRAINING TOTALS:					

WORKOUT REMINDER:

_____

_____

_____

_____

_____

COMMENTS:

OTHER·GROUP EXERCISE   STRETCHING/WARMUP: yes ❑ no ❑

Time	Exercise Type	Minutes	Cal. Burned
OTHER·GROUP EXERCISE TOTALS:			

COMMENTS:

DAILY GOAL(S) _____

_____

_____

**DAILY GOALS
ACHIEVED**

FLEXIBILITY · RELAXATION · MEDITATION

Activity Performed	Minutes
FLEXIBILITY · RELAXATION · MEDITATION TOTALS:	
COMMENTS:	

NUTRITIONAL INTAKE

Food Item	amt.	cal.	fat gms	protein gms	carbs gms	fiber gms
BREAKFAST:						
LUNCH:						
DINNER:						
SNACKS:						
INTAKE TOTALS:						

VITAMINS & SUPPLEMENTS

Type: _____

Qty: _____

Type: _____

Qty: _____

Type: _____

Qty: _____

Type: _____

Qty: _____

WATER INTAKE:

OF 8OZ GLASSES

❑ ❑

❑ ❑

❑ ❑

❑ ❑

❑ ❑

COMMENTS · NOTES · PROGRESS

_____

_____

_____

_____

_____

DATE:_____ WEEK#:_____ DAY#:_____   WEIGHT:_____

ENERGY LEVELS: low ☐ med ☐ high ☐

Helpful Tips

Daily Workout Journal

CARDIOVASCULAR EXERCISE   STRETCHING/WARMUP: yes ☐ no ☐

By the time
you feel
thirsty,
your body
has already
become
dehydrated.
Drink water
before you
feel thirsty.

Time	Exercise Type	Minutes	Distance	Pace/ Setting	Cal. Burned
CARDIO EXERCISE TOTALS:					

COMMENTS:

STRENGTH TRAINING   TARGET AREA: upper body ☐ lower body ☐ abs ☐

Exercise Type	Muscle Group	SET 1 Reps/Wt.	SET 2 Reps/Wt.	SET 3 Reps/Wt.	SET 4 Reps/Wt.
STRENGTH TRAINING TOTALS:					

WORKOUT REMINDER:

COMMENTS:

OTHER · GROUP EXERCISE   STRETCHING/WARMUP: yes ☐ no ☐

Time	Exercise Type	Minutes	Cal. Burned
OTHER · GROUP EXERCISE TOTALS:			

COMMENTS:

DAILY GOAL(S) _____

_____

_____

DAILY GOALS
ACHIEVED

FLEXIBILITY · RELAXATION · MEDITATION

Activity Performed	Minutes
FLEXIBILITY · RELAXATION · MEDITATION TOTALS:	
COMMENTS:	

NUTRITIONAL INTAKE

Food Item	amt.	cal.	fat gms	protein gms	carbs gms	fiber gms
BREAKFAST:						
LUNCH:						
DINNER:						
SNACKS:						
INTAKE TOTALS:						

VITAMINS & SUPPLEMENTS

Type: _____

Qty: _____

Type: _____

Qty: _____

Type: _____

Qty: _____

Type: _____

Qty: _____

WATER INTAKE:

OF 8OZ GLASSES

❏ ❏

❏ ❏

❏ ❏

❏ ❏

❏ ❏

COMMENTS · NOTES · PROGRESS

_____

_____

_____

_____

_____

DATE:_____ WEEK#:_____ DAY#:_____ WEIGHT:_____

ENERGY LEVELS: low ☐ med ☐ high ☐

Helpful Tips

Daily Workout Journal

Eating lean protein such as fish and turkey will encourage the building of lean muscle mass while helping you feel full longer.

CARDIOVASCULAR EXERCISE   STRETCHING/WARMUP: yes ☐ no ☐

Time	Exercise Type	Minutes	Distance	Pace/Setting	Cal. Burned
CARDIO EXERCISE TOTALS:					

COMMENTS:

STRENGTH TRAINING   TARGET AREA: upper body ☐ lower body ☐ abs ☐

Exercise Type	Muscle Group	SET 1 Reps/Wt.	SET 2 Reps/Wt.	SET 3 Reps/Wt.	SET 4 Reps/Wt.
STRENGTH TRAINING TOTALS:					

WORKOUT REMINDER:

_____
_____
_____
_____
_____
_____
_____
_____
_____

COMMENTS:

OTHER·GROUP EXERCISE   STRETCHING/WARMUP: yes ☐ no ☐

Time	Exercise Type	Minutes	Cal. Burned
OTHER·GROUP EXERCISE TOTALS:			

COMMENTS:

DAILY GOAL(S) _____

_____

_____

**DAILY GOALS
ACHIEVED**

FLEXIBILITY · RELAXATION · MEDITATION

Activity Performed	Minutes
FLEXIBILITY · RELAXATION · MEDITATION TOTALS:	
COMMENTS:	

NUTRITIONAL INTAKE

Food Item	amt.	cal.	fat gms	protein gms	carbs gms	fiber gms
BREAKFAST:						
LUNCH:						
DINNER:						
SNACKS:						
INTAKE TOTALS:						

**VITAMINS &
SUPPLEMENTS**

Type: _____

Qty: _____

Type: _____

Qty: _____

Type: _____

Qty: _____

Type: _____

Qty: _____

WATER INTAKE:

OF 8OZ GLASSES

❏ ❏

❏ ❏

❏ ❏

❏ ❏

❏ ❏

COMMENTS · NOTES · PROGRESS

_____

_____

_____

_____

_____

DATE:_____ WEEK#:_____ DAY#:_____   WEIGHT:_____

ENERGY LEVELS: low ❑ med ❑ high ❑

Daily Workout Journal

CARDIOVASCULAR EXERCISE   STRETCHING/WARMUP: yes ❑ no ❑

Eating a
proper
breakfast,
which includes
protein and
complex
carbohydrates,
will provide
your body with
the energy
it will need
throughout
the day as
well as jump-
start your
metabolism.

Time	Exercise Type	Minutes	Distance	Pace/ Setting	Cal. Burned
CARDIO EXERCISE TOTALS:					

COMMENTS:

STRENGTH TRAINING   TARGET AREA: upper body ❑ lower body ❑ abs ❑

Exercise Type	Muscle Group	SET 1 Reps/Wt.	SET 2 Reps/Wt.	SET 3 Reps/Wt.	SET 4 Reps/Wt.
STRENGTH TRAINING TOTALS:					

COMMENTS:

OTHER · GROUP EXERCISE   STRETCHING/WARMUP: yes ❑ no ❑

Time	Exercise Type	Minutes	Cal. Burned
OTHER · GROUP EXERCISE TOTALS:			

COMMENTS:

FLEXIBILITY · RELAXATION · MEDITATION

Activity Performed	Minutes
FLEXIBILITY · RELAXATION · MEDITATION TOTALS:	
COMMENTS:	

NUTRITIONAL INTAKE

Food Item	amt.	cal.	fat gms	protein gms	carbs gms	fiber gms
BREAKFAST:						
LUNCH:						
DINNER:						
SNACKS:						
INTAKE TOTALS:						

VITAMINS & SUPPLEMENTS

Type: _____
Qty: _____

Type: _____
Qty: _____

Type: _____
Qty: _____

Type: _____
Qty: _____

WATER INTAKE:
OF 8oz GLASSES

❏ ❏

❏ ❏

❏ ❏

❏ ❏

❏ ❏

COMMENTS · NOTES · PROGRESS

_____

_____

_____

_____

_____

DATE:_____ WEEK#:_____ DAY#:_____   WEIGHT:_____

Helpful Tips

Daily Workout Journal

Maintaining a
regular eating
schedule will
help your
body digest
food properly.

CARDIOVASCULAR EXERCISE   STRETCHING/WARMUP: yes ☐ no ☐

Time	Exercise Type	Minutes	Distance	Pace/Setting	Cal. Burned
CARDIO EXERCISE TOTALS:					

COMMENTS:

STRENGTH TRAINING   TARGET AREA: upper body ☐ lower body ☐ abs ☐

Exercise Type	Muscle Group	SET 1 Reps/Wt.	SET 2 Reps/Wt.	SET 3 Reps/Wt.	SET 4 Reps/Wt.
STRENGTH TRAINING TOTALS:					

**WORKOUT
REMINDER:**

_____

_____

_____

_____

_____

_____

_____

_____

_____

_____

_____

COMMENTS:

OTHER · GROUP EXERCISE   STRETCHING/WARMUP: yes ☐ no ☐

Time	Exercise Type	Minutes	Cal. Burned
OTHER · GROUP EXERCISE TOTALS:			

COMMENTS:

DAILY GOAL(S) _____

_____

_____

DAILY GOALS
ACHIEVED

FLEXIBILITY · RELAXATION · MEDITATION

Activity Performed	Minutes
FLEXIBILITY · RELAXATION · MEDITATION TOTALS:	
COMMENTS:	

NUTRITIONAL INTAKE

Food Item	amt.	cal.	fat gms	protein gms	carbs gms	fiber gms
BREAKFAST:						
LUNCH:						
DINNER:						
SNACKS:						
INTAKE TOTALS:						

VITAMINS &
SUPPLEMENTS

Type: _____
Qty: _____

Type: _____
Qty: _____

Type: _____
Qty: _____

Type: _____
Qty: _____

WATER INTAKE:
OF 8OZ GLASSES

❑ ❑
❑ ❑
❑ ❑
❑ ❑
❑ ❑

COMMENTS · NOTES · PROGRESS

_____

_____

_____

_____

_____

ENERGY LEVELS: low ❏ med ❏ high ❏

Helpful Tips

Daily Workout Journal

Eating large
amounts of
food close to
bedtime can
interfere with
your body's
digestion;
metabolism
slows and
excess
calories are
stored as fat.

CARDIOVASCULAR EXERCISE   STRETCHING/WARMUP: yes ❏ no ❏

Time	Exercise Type	Minutes	Distance	Pace/ Setting	Cal. Burned
CARDIO EXERCISE TOTALS:					

COMMENTS:

STRENGTH TRAINING   TARGET AREA: upper body ❏ lower body ❏ abs ❏

Exercise Type	Muscle Group	SET 1 Reps/Wt.	SET 2 Reps/Wt.	SET 3 Reps/Wt.	SET 4 Reps/Wt.
STRENGTH TRAINING TOTALS:					

COMMENTS:

WORKOUT REMINDER:

_____

_____

_____

_____

_____

_____

_____

_____

_____

_____

OTHER · GROUP EXERCISE   STRETCHING/WARMUP: yes ❏ no ❏

Time	Exercise Type	Minutes	Cal. Burned
OTHER · GROUP EXERCISE TOTALS:			

COMMENTS:

DAILY GOAL(S)_____

_____

_____

**DAILY GOALS
ACHIEVED**

FLEXIBILITY · RELAXATION · MEDITATION

Activity Performed	Minutes
FLEXIBILITY · RELAXATION · MEDITATION TOTALS:	
COMMENTS:	

NUTRITIONAL INTAKE

Food Item	amt.	cal.	fat gms	protein gms	carbs gms	fiber gms
BREAKFAST:						
LUNCH:						
DINNER:						
SNACKS:						
INTAKE TOTALS:						

**VITAMINS &
SUPPLEMENTS**

Type:_____
Qty:_____

Type:_____
Qty:_____

Type:_____
Qty:_____

Type:_____
Qty:_____

WATER INTAKE:

OF 8OZ GLASSES

❑ ❑

❑ ❑

❑ ❑

❑ ❑

❑ ❑

COMMENTS · NOTES · PROGRESS

_____

_____

_____

_____

_____

DATE:_____ WEEK#:_____ DAY#:_____ WEIGHT:_____

Helpful Tips

Daily Workout Journal

CARDIOVASCULAR EXERCISE   STRETCHING/WARMUP: yes ☐ no ☐

Time	Exercise Type	Minutes	Distance	Pace/Setting	Cal. Burned
CARDIO EXERCISE TOTALS:					

COMMENTS:

STRENGTH TRAINING   TARGET AREA: upper body ☐ lower body ☐ abs ☐

Exercise Type	Muscle Group	SET 1 Reps/Wt.	SET 2 Reps/Wt.	SET 3 Reps/Wt.	SET 4 Reps/Wt.
STRENGTH TRAINING TOTALS:					

WORKOUT REMINDER:

_____

_____

_____

_____

_____

COMMENTS:

OTHER · GROUP EXERCISE   STRETCHING/WARMUP: yes ☐ no ☐

Time	Exercise Type	Minutes	Cal. Burned
OTHER · GROUP EXERCISE TOTALS:			

_____

_____

_____

_____

COMMENTS:

DAILY GOAL(S) _____

_____

_____

DAILY GOALS ACHIEVED

FLEXIBILITY · RELAXATION · MEDITATION

Activity Performed	Minutes
FLEXIBILITY · RELAXATION · MEDITATION TOTALS:	
COMMENTS:	

NUTRITIONAL INTAKE

Food Item	amt.	cal.	fat gms	protein gms	carbs gms	fiber gms
BREAKFAST:						
LUNCH:						
DINNER:						
SNACKS:						
INTAKE TOTALS:						

VITAMINS & SUPPLEMENTS

Type: _____

Qty: _____

Type: _____

Qty: _____

Type: _____

Qty: _____

Type: _____

Qty: _____

Type: _____

Qty: _____

WATER INTAKE:

OF 8OZ GLASSES

❑ ❑

❑ ❑

❑ ❑

❑ ❑

❑ ❑

COMMENTS · NOTES · PROGRESS

_____

_____

_____

_____

_____

ENERGY LEVELS: low ☐ med ☐ high ☐

Daily Workout Journal

CARDIOVASCULAR EXERCISE STRETCHING/WARMUP: yes ☐ no ☐

Time	Exercise Type	Minutes	Distance	Pace/ Setting	Cal. Burned
CARDIO EXERCISE TOTALS:					

COMMENTS:

STRENGTH TRAINING TARGET AREA: upper body ☐ lower body ☐ abs ☐

Exercise Type	Muscle Group	SET 1 Reps/Wt.	SET 2 Reps/Wt.	SET 3 Reps/Wt.	SET 4 Reps/Wt.
STRENGTH TRAINING TOTALS:					

COMMENTS:

OTHER · GROUP EXERCISE STRETCHING/WARMUP: yes ☐ no ☐

Time	Exercise Type	Minutes	Cal. Burned
OTHER · GROUP EXERCISE TOTALS:			

COMMENTS:

DAILY GOAL(S) _____

_____

_____

FLEXIBILITY · RELAXATION · MEDITATION

Activity Performed	Minutes
FLEXIBILITY · RELAXATION · MEDITATION TOTALS:	
COMMENTS:	

NUTRITIONAL INTAKE

Food Item	amt.	cal.	fat gms	protein gms	carbs gms	fiber gms
BREAKFAST:						
LUNCH:						
DINNER:						
SNACKS:						
INTAKE TOTALS:						

**VITAMINS &
SUPPLEMENTS**

Type: _____
Qty: _____

Type: _____
Qty: _____

Type: _____
Qty: _____

Type: _____
Qty: _____

WATER INTAKE:

OF 8OZ GLASSES

❑ ❑

❑ ❑

❑ ❑

❑ ❑

❑ ❑

COMMENTS · NOTES · PROGRESS

_____

_____

_____

_____

_____

DATE:_____ WEEK#:_____ DAY#:_____   WEIGHT:_____

ENERGY LEVELS: low ☐ med ☐ high ☐

Daily Workout Journal

CARDIOVASCULAR EXERCISE   STRETCHING/WARMUP: yes ☐ no ☐

Hunger
sensations
may actually
mean you
need water.
If you've
recently
eaten and
start feeling
hungry,
drinking
a glass of
water may
alleviate your
hunger.

Time	Exercise Type	Minutes	Distance	Pace/Setting	Cal. Burned
CARDIO EXERCISE TOTALS:					

COMMENTS:

STRENGTH TRAINING   TARGET AREA: upper body ☐ lower body ☐ abs ☐

Exercise Type	Muscle Group	SET 1 Reps/Wt.	SET 2 Reps/Wt.	SET 3 Reps/Wt.	SET 4 Reps/Wt.
STRENGTH TRAINING TOTALS:					

COMMENTS:

OTHER · GROUP EXERCISE   STRETCHING/WARMUP: yes ☐ no ☐

Time	Exercise Type	Minutes	Cal. Burned
OTHER · GROUP EXERCISE TOTALS:			

COMMENTS:

DAILY GOAL(S) _____

_____

_____

FLEXIBILITY · RELAXATION · MEDITATION

Activity Performed	Minutes
FLEXIBILITY · RELAXATION · MEDITATION TOTALS:	
COMMENTS:	

NUTRITIONAL INTAKE

Food Item	amt.	cal.	fat gms	protein gms	carbs gms	fiber gms
BREAKFAST:						
LUNCH:						
DINNER:						
SNACKS:						
INTAKE TOTALS:						

VITAMINS & SUPPLEMENTS

Type: _____
Qty: _____

Type: _____
Qty: _____

Type: _____
Qty: _____

Type: _____
Qty: _____

WATER INTAKE:
OF 8OZ GLASSES

❑ ❑
❑ ❑
❑ ❑
❑ ❑
❑ ❑

COMMENTS · NOTES · PROGRESS

_____

_____

_____

_____

_____

DATE:_____ WEEK#:_____ DAY#:_____   WEIGHT:_____

Helpful Tips

Daily Workout Journal

Skipping
meals or
eating too
little at a
meal can
slow your
metabolism.

CARDIOVASCULAR EXERCISE   STRETCHING/WARMUP: yes ❏ no ❏

Time	Exercise Type	Minutes	Distance	Pace/ Setting	Cal. Burned
CARDIO EXERCISE TOTALS:					

COMMENTS:

STRENGTH TRAINING   TARGET AREA: upper body ❏ lower body ❏ abs ❏

Exercise Type	Muscle Group	SET 1 Reps/Wt.	SET 2 Reps/Wt.	SET 3 Reps/Wt.	SET 4 Reps/Wt.
STRENGTH TRAINING TOTALS:					

COMMENTS:

WORKOUT REMINDER:

_____

_____

_____

_____

_____

_____

_____

_____

_____

_____

OTHER · GROUP EXERCISE   STRETCHING/WARMUP: yes ❏ no ❏

Time	Exercise Type	Minutes	Cal. Burned
OTHER · GROUP EXERCISE TOTALS:			

COMMENTS:

DAILY GOAL(S) _____

_____

_____

**DAILY GOALS
ACHIEVED**

FLEXIBILITY · RELAXATION · MEDITATION

Activity Performed	Minutes
FLEXIBILITY · RELAXATION · MEDITATION TOTALS:	
COMMENTS:	

NUTRITIONAL INTAKE

Food Item	amt.	cal.	fat gms	protein gms	carbs gms	fiber gms
BREAKFAST:						
LUNCH:						
DINNER:						
SNACKS:						
INTAKE TOTALS:						

**VITAMINS &
SUPPLEMENTS**

Type: _____
Qty: _____

Type: _____
Qty: _____

Type: _____
Qty: _____

Type: _____
Qty: _____

WATER INTAKE:

OF 8OZ GLASSES

❑ ❑

❑ ❑

❑ ❑

❑ ❑

❑ ❑

COMMENTS · NOTES · PROGRESS

_____

_____

_____

_____

_____

_____

ENERGY LEVELS: low ☐   med ☐   high ☐

Helpful Tips

Daily Workout Journal

CARDIOVASCULAR EXERCISE   STRETCHING/WARMUP: yes ☐ no ☐

If you do not
get adequate
rest, your body
may attempt
to compensate
for its fatigue
by craving
sugar and
carbohydrates
that provide a
quick burst of
energy.

Time	Exercise Type	Minutes	Distance	Pace/ Setting	Cal. Burned
CARDIO EXERCISE TOTALS:					

COMMENTS:

STRENGTH TRAINING   TARGET AREA: upper body ☐ lower body ☐ abs ☐

Exercise Type	Muscle Group	SET 1 Reps/Wt.	SET 2 Reps/Wt.	SET 3 Reps/Wt.	SET 4 Reps/Wt.
STRENGTH TRAINING TOTALS:					

**WORKOUT
REMINDER:**

_____

_____

_____

_____

_____

COMMENTS:

OTHER · GROUP EXERCISE   STRETCHING/WARMUP: yes ☐ no ☐

_____

_____

Time	Exercise Type	Minutes	Cal. Burned
OTHER · GROUP EXERCISE TOTALS:			

_____

_____

COMMENTS:

DAILY GOAL(S) _____

_____

_____

DAILY GOALS
ACHIEVED

FLEXIBILITY · RELAXATION · MEDITATION

Activity Performed	Minutes
FLEXIBILITY · RELAXATION · MEDITATION TOTALS:	

COMMENTS:

NUTRITIONAL INTAKE

Food Item	amt.	cal.	fat gms	protein gms	carbs gms	fiber gms
BREAKFAST:						
LUNCH:						
DINNER:						
SNACKS:						
INTAKE TOTALS:						

VITAMINS & SUPPLEMENTS

Type: _____
Qty: _____

Type: _____
Qty: _____

Type: _____
Qty: _____

Type: _____
Qty: _____

WATER INTAKE:
OF 8OZ GLASSES

❏ ❏
❏ ❏
❏ ❏
❏ ❏
❏ ❏

COMMENTS · NOTES · PROGRESS

_____

_____

_____

_____

_____

DATE:_____ WEEK#:_____ DAY#:_____ WEIGHT:_____

Helpful Tips

Daily Workout Journal

When eating out, avoiding sweets and chips will keep you from consuming empty calories.

CARDIOVASCULAR EXERCISE STRETCHING/WARMUP: yes ❑ no ❑

Time	Exercise Type	Minutes	Distance	Pace/ Setting	Cal. Burned
CARDIO EXERCISE TOTALS:					

COMMENTS:

STRENGTH TRAINING TARGET AREA: upper body ❑ lower body ❑ abs ❑

Exercise Type	Muscle Group	SET 1 Reps/Wt.	SET 2 Reps/Wt.	SET 3 Reps/Wt.	SET 4 Reps/Wt.
STRENGTH TRAINING TOTALS:					

WORKOUT REMINDER:

_____

_____

_____

_____

_____

_____

_____

_____

_____

_____

COMMENTS:

OTHER · GROUP EXERCISE STRETCHING/WARMUP: yes ❑ no ❑

Time	Exercise Type	Minutes	Cal. Burned
OTHER·GROUP EXERCISE TOTALS:			

COMMENTS:

DAILY GOALS ACHIEVED

FLEXIBILITY · RELAXATION · MEDITATION

Activity Performed	Minutes
FLEXIBILITY · RELAXATION · MEDITATION TOTALS:	
COMMENTS:	

NUTRITIONAL INTAKE

Food Item	amt.	cal.	fat gms	protein gms	carbs gms	fiber gms
BREAKFAST:						
LUNCH:						
DINNER:						
SNACKS:						
INTAKE TOTALS:						

VITAMINS & SUPPLEMENTS

Type: _____
Qty: _____

Type: _____
Qty: _____

Type: _____
Qty: _____

Type: _____
Qty: _____

WATER INTAKE:
OF 8OZ GLASSES

❑ ❑
❑ ❑
❑ ❑
❑ ❑
❑ ❑

COMMENTS · NOTES · PROGRESS

DATE:_____ WEEK#:_____ DAY#:_____   WEIGHT:_____

Helpful Tips   # Daily Workout Journal

When
eating out,
ordering a
soup or salad
will help
you avoid
unhealthy
temptations,
such as
high-calorie
appetizers.

CARDIOVASCULAR EXERCISE   STRETCHING/WARMUP: yes ❑ no ❑

Time	Exercise Type	Minutes	Distance	Pace/ Setting	Cal. Burned
CARDIO EXERCISE TOTALS:					

COMMENTS:

STRENGTH TRAINING   TARGET AREA: upper body ❑ lower body ❑ abs ❑

Exercise Type	Muscle Group	SET 1 Reps/Wt.	SET 2 Reps/Wt.	SET 3 Reps/Wt.	SET 4 Reps/Wt.
STRENGTH TRAINING TOTALS:					

**WORKOUT
REMINDER:**

_____

_____

_____

_____

COMMENTS:

OTHER · GROUP EXERCISE   STRETCHING/WARMUP: yes ❑ no ❑

Time	Exercise Type	Minutes	Cal. Burned
OTHER·GROUP EXERCISE TOTALS:			

COMMENTS:

DAILY GOAL(S) _____

_____

**DAILY GOALS
ACHIEVED**

FLEXIBILITY · RELAXATION · MEDITATION

Activity Performed	Minutes
FLEXIBILITY · RELAXATION · MEDITATION TOTALS:	
COMMENTS:	

NUTRITIONAL INTAKE

Food Item	amt.	cal.	fat gms	protein gms	carbs gms	fiber gms
BREAKFAST:						
LUNCH:						
DINNER:						
SNACKS:						
INTAKE TOTALS:						

VITAMINS & SUPPLEMENTS

Type: _____

Qty: _____

Type: _____

Qty: _____

Type: _____

Qty: _____

Type: _____

Qty: _____

WATER INTAKE:

OF 8OZ GLASSES

❏ ❏

❏ ❏

❏ ❏

❏ ❏

❏ ❏

COMMENTS · NOTES · PROGRESS

_____

_____

_____

_____

_____

DATE:_____ WEEK#:_____ DAY#:_____   WEIGHT:_____

Helpful Tips

Daily Workout Journal

Often, restaurant entrees are large enough for two or three meals. When eating out, be aware of the size of the entree and consider taking part of it home.

CARDIOVASCULAR EXERCISE   STRETCHING/WARMUP: yes ☐ no ☐

Time	Exercise Type	Minutes	Distance	Pace/ Setting	Cal. Burned
CARDIO EXERCISE TOTALS:					

COMMENTS:

STRENGTH TRAINING   TARGET AREA: upper body ☐ lower body ☐ abs ☐

Exercise Type	Muscle Group	SET 1 Reps/Wt.	SET 2 Reps/Wt.	SET 3 Reps/Wt.	SET 4 Reps/Wt.
STRENGTH TRAINING TOTALS:					

WORKOUT REMINDER:

_____

_____

_____

_____

COMMENTS:

OTHER · GROUP EXERCISE   STRETCHING/WARMUP: yes ☐ no ☐

Time	Exercise Type	Minutes	Cal. Burned
OTHER · GROUP EXERCISE TOTALS:			

COMMENTS:

DAILY GOAL(S) _____
_____
_____

DAILY GOALS ACHIEVED

FLEXIBILITY · RELAXATION · MEDITATION

Activity Performed	Minutes
FLEXIBILITY · RELAXATION · MEDITATION TOTALS:	
COMMENTS:	

NUTRITIONAL INTAKE

Food Item	amt.	cal.	fat gms	protein gms	carbs gms	fiber gms
BREAKFAST:						
LUNCH:						
DINNER:						
SNACKS:						
INTAKE TOTALS:						

VITAMINS & SUPPLEMENTS

Type: _____
Qty: _____

Type: _____
Qty: _____

Type: _____
Qty: _____

Type: _____
Qty: _____

WATER INTAKE:
OF 8OZ GLASSES

☐ ☐
☐ ☐
☐ ☐
☐ ☐
☐ ☐

COMMENTS · NOTES · PROGRESS

_____
_____
_____
_____
_____

DATE:_____ WEEK#:_____ DAY#:_____   WEIGHT:_____

ENERGY LEVELS: low ☐ med ☐ high ☐

Daily Workout Journal

Low
carbohydrate
diets deny
the body its
main source
of energy
and reduce
its ability to
metabolize
food, often
resulting in
diminished
weight loss.

CARDIOVASCULAR EXERCISE   STRETCHING/WARMUP: yes ☐ no ☐

Time	Exercise Type	Minutes	Distance	Pace/ Setting	Cal. Burned
CARDIO EXERCISE TOTALS:					

COMMENTS:

STRENGTH TRAINING   TARGET AREA: upper body ☐ lower body ☐ abs ☐

Exercise Type	Muscle Group	SET 1 Reps/Wt.	SET 2 Reps/Wt.	SET 3 Reps/Wt.	SET 4 Reps/Wt.
STRENGTH TRAINING TOTALS:					

**WORKOUT
REMINDER:**

_____
_____
_____
_____
_____
_____
_____
_____
_____

COMMENTS:

OTHER · GROUP EXERCISE   STRETCHING/WARMUP: yes ☐ no ☐

Time	Exercise Type	Minutes	Cal. Burned
OTHER · GROUP EXERCISE TOTALS:			

COMMENTS:

I DID IT!

DAILY GOALS
ACHIEVED

FLEXIBILITY · RELAXATION · MEDITATION

Activity Performed	Minutes
FLEXIBILITY · RELAXATION · MEDITATION TOTALS:	
COMMENTS:	

NUTRITIONAL INTAKE

Food Item	amt.	cal.	fat gms	protein gms	carbs gms	fiber gms
BREAKFAST:						
LUNCH:						
DINNER:						
SNACKS:						
INTAKE TOTALS:						

VITAMINS & SUPPLEMENTS

Type: _____
Qty: _____

Type: _____
Qty: _____

Type: _____
Qty: _____

Type: _____
Qty: _____

WATER INTAKE:

OF 8OZ GLASSES

❑ ❑
❑ ❑
❑ ❑
❑ ❑
❑ ❑

COMMENTS · NOTES · PROGRESS

DATE:_____ WEEK#:_____ DAY#:_____ WEIGHT:_____

Helpful Tips

Daily Workout Journal

CARDIOVASCULAR EXERCISE   STRETCHING/WARMUP: yes ❑ no ❑

Time	Exercise Type	Minutes	Distance	Pace/ Setting	Cal. Burned
CARDIO EXERCISE TOTALS:					

COMMENTS:

STRENGTH TRAINING   TARGET AREA: upper body ❑ lower body ❑ abs ❑

Exercise Type	Muscle Group	SET 1 Reps/Wt.	SET 2 Reps/Wt.	SET 3 Reps/Wt.	SET 4 Reps/Wt.
STRENGTH TRAINING TOTALS:					

WORKOUT REMINDER:

_____

_____

_____

_____

_____

_____

_____

_____

_____

_____

COMMENTS:

OTHER · GROUP EXERCISE   STRETCHING/WARMUP: yes ❑ no ❑

Time	Exercise Type	Minutes	Cal. Burned
OTHER · GROUP EXERCISE TOTALS:			

COMMENTS:

DAILY GOAL(S) _____

_____

_____

**DAILY GOALS
ACHIEVED**

FLEXIBILITY · RELAXATION · MEDITATION

Activity Performed	Minutes
FLEXIBILITY · RELAXATION · MEDITATION TOTALS:	
COMMENTS:	

NUTRITIONAL INTAKE

Food Item	amt.	cal.	fat gms	protein gms	carbs gms	fiber gms
BREAKFAST:						
LUNCH:						
DINNER:						
SNACKS:						
INTAKE TOTALS:						

**VITAMINS &
SUPPLEMENTS**

Type: _____

Qty: _____

Type: _____

Qty: _____

Type: _____

Qty: _____

Type: _____

Qty: _____

WATER INTAKE:

OF 8OZ GLASSES

❑ ❑

❑ ❑

❑ ❑

❑ ❑

❑ ❑

COMMENTS · NOTES · PROGRESS

_____

_____

_____

_____

_____

_____

ENERGY LEVELS: low ☐   med ☐   high ☐

Daily Workout Journal

CARDIOVASCULAR EXERCISE   STRETCHING/WARMUP: yes ☐ no ☐

Time	Exercise Type	Minutes	Distance	Pace/Setting	Cal. Burned
CARDIO EXERCISE TOTALS:					

COMMENTS:

STRENGTH TRAINING   TARGET AREA: upper body ☐ lower body ☐ abs ☐

Exercise Type	Muscle Group	SET 1 Reps/Wt.	SET 2 Reps/Wt.	SET 3 Reps/Wt.	SET 4 Reps/Wt.
STRENGTH TRAINING TOTALS:					

COMMENTS:

OTHER · GROUP EXERCISE   STRETCHING/WARMUP: yes ☐ no ☐

Time	Exercise Type	Minutes	Cal. Burned
OTHER · GROUP EXERCISE TOTALS:			

COMMENTS:

FLEXIBILITY · RELAXATION · MEDITATION

Activity Performed	Minutes
FLEXIBILITY · RELAXATION · MEDITATION TOTALS:	

COMMENTS:

NUTRITIONAL INTAKE

Food Item	amt.	cal.	fat gms	protein gms	carbs gms	fiber gms
BREAKFAST:						
LUNCH:						
DINNER:						
SNACKS:						
INTAKE TOTALS:						

VITAMINS & SUPPLEMENTS

Type:
Qty:

Type:
Qty:

Type:
Qty:

Type:
Qty:

WATER INTAKE:
OF 8OZ GLASSES

❏ ❏
❏ ❏
❏ ❏
❏ ❏
❏ ❏

COMMENTS · NOTES · PROGRESS

DATE:_____ WEEK#:_____ DAY#:_____ WEIGHT:_____

Helpful Tips

Daily Workout Journal

Although caffeine is a stimulant, it can leave you feeling weak once its effects wear off. Avoid using caffeinated beverages for quick burst of energy. More than 2 cups per day can interfere with sleep and make you prone to withdrawal symptoms if your source of caffeine is cut off.

WORKOUT REMINDER:

_____
_____
_____
_____
_____
_____
_____
_____
_____
_____
_____
_____

CARDIOVASCULAR EXERCISE   STRETCHING/WARMUP: yes ☐ no ☐

Time	Exercise Type	Minutes	Distance	Pace/ Setting	Cal. Burned
CARDIO EXERCISE TOTALS:					

COMMENTS:

STRENGTH TRAINING   TARGET AREA: upper body ☐ lower body ☐ abs ☐

Exercise Type	Muscle Group	SET 1 Reps/Wt.	SET 2 Reps/Wt.	SET 3 Reps/Wt.	SET 4 Reps/Wt.
STRENGTH TRAINING TOTALS:					

COMMENTS:

OTHER·GROUP EXERCISE   STRETCHING/WARMUP: yes ☐ no ☐

Time	Exercise Type	Minutes	Cal. Burned
OTHER·GROUP EXERCISE TOTALS:			

COMMENTS:

DAILY GOAL(S) _____

_____

_____

**DAILY GOALS
ACHIEVED**

FLEXIBILITY · RELAXATION · MEDITATION

Activity Performed	Minutes
FLEXIBILITY · RELAXATION · MEDITATION TOTALS:	

COMMENTS:

NUTRITIONAL INTAKE

Food Item	amt.	cal.	fat gms	protein gms	carbs gms	fiber gms
BREAKFAST:						
LUNCH:						
DINNER:						
SNACKS:						
INTAKE TOTALS:						

**VITAMINS &
SUPPLEMENTS**

Type: _____

Qty: _____

Type: _____

Qty: _____

Type: _____

Qty: _____

Type: _____

Qty: _____

WATER INTAKE:

OF 8OZ GLASSES

❏ ❏
❏ ❏
❏ ❏
❏ ❏
❏ ❏

COMMENTS · NOTES · PROGRESS

_____

_____

_____

_____

_____

DATE:_____ WEEK#:_____ DAY#:_____   WEIGHT:_____

ENERGY LEVELS: low ☐ med ☐ high ☐

Daily Workout Journal

Good shoes
that fit
properly
should feel
comfortable
right away.
Never
purchase
athletic shoes
with the idea
that they
will fit better
once you
break them
in.

CARDIOVASCULAR EXERCISE   STRETCHING/WARMUP: yes ☐ no ☐

Time	Exercise Type	Minutes	Distance	Pace/ Setting	Cal. Burned
CARDIO EXERCISE TOTALS:					

COMMENTS:

STRENGTH TRAINING   TARGET AREA: upper body ☐ lower body ☐ abs ☐

Exercise Type	Muscle Group	SET 1 Reps/Wt.	SET 2 Reps/Wt.	SET 3 Reps/Wt.	SET 4 Reps/Wt.
STRENGTH TRAINING TOTALS:					

COMMENTS:

OTHER · GROUP EXERCISE   STRETCHING/WARMUP: yes ☐ no ☐

Time	Exercise Type	Minutes	Cal. Burned
OTHER · GROUP EXERCISE TOTALS:			

COMMENTS:

DAILY GOAL(S) _____

_____

_____

I DID IT!

DAILY GOALS ACHIEVED

FLEXIBILITY · RELAXATION · MEDITATION

Activity Performed	Minutes
FLEXIBILITY · RELAXATION · MEDITATION TOTALS:	
COMMENTS:	

NUTRITIONAL INTAKE

Food Item	amt.	cal.	fat gms	protein gms	carbs gms	fiber gms
BREAKFAST:						
LUNCH:						
DINNER:						
SNACKS:						
INTAKE TOTALS:						

VITAMINS & SUPPLEMENTS

Type: _____
Qty: _____

Type: _____
Qty: _____

Type: _____
Qty: _____

Type: _____
Qty: _____

WATER INTAKE:
OF 8oz GLASSES

❑ ❑

❑ ❑

❑ ❑

❑ ❑

❑ ❑

COMMENTS · NOTES · PROGRESS

_____

_____

_____

_____

_____

ENERGY LEVELS: low ☐ med ☐ high ☐

Helpful Tips

Daily Workout Journal

Running shoes should have a ½" space between the end of the shoe and the end of your longest toe. Your heel should not move around in the shoe.

CARDIOVASCULAR EXERCISE   STRETCHING/WARMUP: yes ☐ no ☐

Time	Exercise Type	Minutes	Distance	Pace/Setting	Cal. Burned
CARDIO EXERCISE TOTALS:					

COMMENTS:

STRENGTH TRAINING   TARGET AREA: upper body ☐ lower body ☐ abs ☐

Exercise Type	Muscle Group	SET 1 Reps/Wt.	SET 2 Reps/Wt.	SET 3 Reps/Wt.	SET 4 Reps/Wt.
STRENGTH TRAINING TOTALS:					

WORKOUT REMINDER:

COMMENTS:

OTHER · GROUP EXERCISE   STRETCHING/WARMUP: yes ☐ no ☐

Time	Exercise Type	Minutes	Cal. Burned
OTHER · GROUP EXERCISE TOTALS:			

COMMENTS:

DAILY GOAL(S)_____

_____

_____

**DAILY GOALS
ACHIEVED**

FLEXIBILITY · RELAXATION · MEDITATION

Activity Performed	Minutes
FLEXIBILITY · RELAXATION · MEDITATION TOTALS:	
COMMENTS:	

NUTRITIONAL INTAKE

Food Item	amt.	cal.	fat gms	protein gms	carbs gms	fiber gms
BREAKFAST:						
LUNCH:						
DINNER:						
SNACKS:						
INTAKE TOTALS:						

**VITAMINS &
SUPPLEMENTS**

Type:_____
Qty:_____

Type:_____
Qty:_____

Type:_____
Qty:_____

Type:_____
Qty:_____

WATER INTAKE:

OF 8OZ GLASSES

❑ ❑
❑ ❑
❑ ❑
❑ ❑
❑ ❑

COMMENTS · NOTES · PROGRESS

_____

_____

_____

_____

_____

DATE:_____ WEEK#:_____ DAY#:_____   WEIGHT:_____

Helpful Tips

Daily Workout Journal

Warm-up exercises help your workouts by sending nutrients and oxygen to muscles that are about to be exercised.

CARDIOVASCULAR EXERCISE   STRETCHING/WARMUP: yes ☐ no ☐

Time	Exercise Type	Minutes	Distance	Pace/ Setting	Cal. Burned
CARDIO EXERCISE TOTALS:					

COMMENTS:

STRENGTH TRAINING   TARGET AREA: upper body ☐ lower body ☐ abs ☐

Exercise Type	Muscle Group	SET 1 Reps/Wt.	SET 2 Reps/Wt.	SET 3 Reps/Wt.	SET 4 Reps/Wt.
STRENGTH TRAINING TOTALS:					

WORKOUT REMINDER:

_____

_____

_____

_____

COMMENTS:

OTHER · GROUP EXERCISE   STRETCHING/WARMUP: yes ☐ no ☐

Time	Exercise Type	Minutes	Cal. Burned
OTHER · GROUP EXERCISE TOTALS:			

COMMENTS:

DAILY GOAL(S) _____

_____

_____

**DAILY GOALS
ACHIEVED**

FLEXIBILITY · RELAXATION · MEDITATION

Activity Performed	Minutes
FLEXIBILITY · RELAXATION · MEDITATION TOTALS:	
COMMENTS:	

NUTRITIONAL INTAKE

Food Item	amt.	cal.	fat gms	protein gms	carbs gms	fiber gms
BREAKFAST:						
LUNCH:						
DINNER:						
SNACKS:						
INTAKE TOTALS:						

**VITAMINS &
SUPPLEMENTS**

Type: _____
Qty: _____

Type: _____
Qty: _____

Type: _____
Qty: _____

Type: _____
Qty: _____

WATER INTAKE:

OF 8oz GLASSES

❑ ❑

❑ ❑

❑ ❑

❑ ❑

❑ ❑

COMMENTS · NOTES · PROGRESS

_____

_____

_____

_____

_____

ENERGY LEVELS: low ☐ med ☐ high ☐

Helpful Tips

Daily Workout Journal

Keeping your workouts light during the first week of a body-building program allows you to focus on form and proper body mechanics. Only after you feel comfortable should you slowly work up to heavier weights.

CARDIOVASCULAR EXERCISE   STRETCHING/WARMUP: yes ☐ no ☐

Time	Exercise Type	Minutes	Distance	Pace/Setting	Cal. Burned
CARDIO EXERCISE TOTALS:					

COMMENTS:

STRENGTH TRAINING   TARGET AREA: upper body ☐ lower body ☐ abs ☐

Exercise Type	Muscle Group	SET 1 Reps/Wt.	SET 2 Reps/Wt.	SET 3 Reps/Wt.	SET 4 Reps/Wt.
STRENGTH TRAINING TOTALS:					

WORKOUT REMINDER:

_____

_____

_____

_____

_____

COMMENTS:

OTHER · GROUP EXERCISE   STRETCHING/WARMUP: yes ☐ no ☐

Time	Exercise Type	Minutes	Cal. Burned
OTHER · GROUP EXERCISE TOTALS:			

COMMENTS:

DAILY GOAL(S) _____

_____

_____

**DAILY GOALS
ACHIEVED**

FLEXIBILITY · RELAXATION · MEDITATION

Activity Performed	Minutes
FLEXIBILITY · RELAXATION · MEDITATION TOTALS:	
COMMENTS:	

NUTRITIONAL INTAKE

Food Item	amt.	cal.	fat gms	protein gms	carbs gms	fiber gms
BREAKFAST:						
LUNCH:						
DINNER:						
SNACKS:						
INTAKE TOTALS:						

**VITAMINS &
SUPPLEMENTS**

Type: _____

Qty: _____

Type: _____

Qty: _____

Type: _____

Qty: _____

Type: _____

Qty: _____

WATER INTAKE:

OF 8OZ GLASSES

❏ ❏

❏ ❏

❏ ❏

❏ ❏

❏ ❏

COMMENTS · NOTES · PROGRESS

_____

_____

_____

_____

_____

_____

ENERGY LEVELS: low ☐ med ☐ high ☐

Daily Workout Journal

Improper weight training form will fail to engage muscles properly and may limit progress. Maintain proper body mechanics and never sacrifice form in order to add more weight or repetitions.

CARDIOVASCULAR EXERCISE   STRETCHING/WARMUP: yes ☐ no ☐

Time	Exercise Type	Minutes	Distance	Pace/ Setting	Cal. Burned
CARDIO EXERCISE TOTALS:					

COMMENTS:

STRENGTH TRAINING   TARGET AREA: upper body ☐ lower body ☐ abs ☐

Exercise Type	Muscle Group	SET 1 Reps/Wt.	SET 2 Reps/Wt.	SET 3 Reps/Wt.	SET 4 Reps/Wt.
STRENGTH TRAINING TOTALS:					

WORKOUT REMINDER:

_____

_____

_____

_____

_____

COMMENTS:

OTHER · GROUP EXERCISE   STRETCHING/WARMUP: yes ☐ no ☐

Time	Exercise Type	Minutes	Cal. Burned
OTHER · GROUP EXERCISE TOTALS:			

_____

_____

_____

_____

_____

COMMENTS:

DAILY GOAL(S) _____

_____

_____

DAILY GOALS
ACHIEVED

FLEXIBILITY · RELAXATION · MEDITATION

Activity Performed	Minutes
FLEXIBILITY · RELAXATION · MEDITATION TOTALS:	
COMMENTS:	

NUTRITIONAL INTAKE

Food Item	amt.	cal.	fat gms	protein gms	carbs gms	fiber gms
BREAKFAST:						
LUNCH:						
DINNER:						
SNACKS:						
INTAKE TOTALS:						

VITAMINS & SUPPLEMENTS

Type: _____
Qty: _____

Type: _____
Qty: _____

Type: _____
Qty: _____

Type: _____
Qty: _____

WATER INTAKE:

OF 8OZ GLASSES

❑ ❑

❑ ❑

❑ ❑

❑ ❑

❑ ❑

COMMENTS · NOTES · PROGRESS

_____

_____

_____

_____

_____

_____

DATE:_____ WEEK#:_____ DAY#:_____   WEIGHT:_____

Helpful Tips   # Daily Workout Journal

Manipulating
the number
of sets,
repetitions,
weight, and
the rest
periods will
help you
reach personal
fitness goals.

CARDIOVASCULAR EXERCISE   STRETCHING/WARMUP: yes ❑ no ❑

Time	Exercise Type	Minutes	Distance	Pace/Setting	Cal. Burned
CARDIO EXERCISE TOTALS:					

COMMENTS:

STRENGTH TRAINING   TARGET AREA: upper body ❑ lower body ❑ abs ❑

Exercise Type	Muscle Group	SET 1 Reps/Wt.	SET 2 Reps/Wt.	SET 3 Reps/Wt.	SET 4 Reps/Wt.
STRENGTH TRAINING TOTALS:					

COMMENTS:

**WORKOUT
REMINDER:**

_____

_____

_____

_____

_____

_____

_____

_____

_____

_____

OTHER · GROUP EXERCISE   STRETCHING/WARMUP: yes ❑ no ❑

Time	Exercise Type	Minutes	Cal. Burned
OTHER · GROUP EXERCISE TOTALS:			

COMMENTS:

DAILY GOAL(S)_____

_____

DAILY GOALS
ACHIEVED

FLEXIBILITY · RELAXATION · MEDITATION

Activity Performed	Minutes
FLEXIBILITY · RELAXATION · MEDITATION TOTALS:	
COMMENTS:	

NUTRITIONAL INTAKE

Food Item	amt.	cal.	fat gms	protein gms	carbs gms	fiber gms
BREAKFAST:						
LUNCH:						
DINNER:						
SNACKS:						
INTAKE TOTALS:						

VITAMINS & SUPPLEMENTS

Type:_____

Qty:_____

Type:_____

Qty:_____

Type:_____

Qty:_____

Type:_____

Qty:_____

WATER INTAKE:
OF 8OZ GLASSES

❏ ❏

❏ ❏

❏ ❏

❏ ❏

❏ ❏

COMMENTS · NOTES · PROGRESS

_____

_____

_____

_____

_____

_____

ENERGY LEVELS: low ☐ med ☐ high ☐

Helpful Tips

Daily Workout Journal

Always listen to your body, especially when strength training. Stop immediately if you feel dizzy or think that you might have injured anything.

CARDIOVASCULAR EXERCISE STRETCHING/WARMUP: yes ☐ no ☐

Time	Exercise Type	Minutes	Distance	Pace/ Setting	Cal. Burned
CARDIO EXERCISE TOTALS:					

COMMENTS:

STRENGTH TRAINING TARGET AREA: upper body ☐ lower body ☐ abs ☐

Exercise Type	Muscle Group	SET 1 Reps/Wt.	SET 2 Reps/Wt.	SET 3 Reps/Wt.	SET 4 Reps/Wt.
STRENGTH TRAINING TOTALS:					

WORKOUT REMINDER:

_____

_____

_____

_____

COMMENTS:

OTHER · GROUP EXERCISE STRETCHING/WARMUP: yes ☐ no ☐

Time	Exercise Type	Minutes	Cal. Burned
OTHER · GROUP EXERCISE TOTALS:			

COMMENTS:

DAILY GOALS
ACHIEVED

FLEXIBILITY · RELAXATION · MEDITATION

Activity Performed	Minutes
FLEXIBILITY · RELAXATION · MEDITATION TOTALS:	
COMMENTS:	

NUTRITIONAL INTAKE

Food Item	amt.	cal.	fat gms	protein gms	carbs gms	fiber gms
BREAKFAST:						
LUNCH:						
DINNER:						
SNACKS:						
INTAKE TOTALS:						

VITAMINS & SUPPLEMENTS

Type:_____
Qty:_____

Type:_____
Qty:_____

Type:_____
Qty:_____

Type:_____
Qty:_____

WATER INTAKE:
OF 8OZ GLASSES

❑ ❑
❑ ❑
❑ ❑
❑ ❑
❑ ❑

COMMENTS · NOTES · PROGRESS

WEIGHT:_____

ENERGY LEVELS: low ☐ med ☐ high ☐

Helpful Tips

Daily Workout Journal

Limit strength training sessions to one hour or less.

CARDIOVASCULAR EXERCISE   STRETCHING/WARMUP: yes ☐ no ☐

Time	Exercise Type	Minutes	Distance	Pace/ Setting	Cal. Burned
CARDIO EXERCISE TOTALS:					

COMMENTS:

STRENGTH TRAINING   TARGET AREA: upper body ☐ lower body ☐ abs ☐

Exercise Type	Muscle Group	SET 1 Reps/Wt.	SET 2 Reps/Wt.	SET 3 Reps/Wt.	SET 4 Reps/Wt.
STRENGTH TRAINING TOTALS:					

WORKOUT REMINDER:

COMMENTS:

OTHER · GROUP EXERCISE   STRETCHING/WARMUP: yes ☐ no ☐

Time	Exercise Type	Minutes	Cal. Burned
OTHER · GROUP EXERCISE TOTALS:			

COMMENTS:

DAILY GOAL(S) _____

_____

_____

**DAILY GOALS
ACHIEVED**

FLEXIBILITY · RELAXATION · MEDITATION

Activity Performed	Minutes
FLEXIBILITY · RELAXATION · MEDITATION TOTALS:	
COMMENTS:	

NUTRITIONAL INTAKE

Food Item	amt.	cal.	fat gms	protein gms	carbs gms	fiber gms
BREAKFAST:						
LUNCH:						
DINNER:						
SNACKS:						
INTAKE TOTALS:						

VITAMINS & SUPPLEMENTS

Type: _____

Qty: _____

Type: _____

Qty: _____

Type: _____

Qty: _____

Type: _____

Qty: _____

WATER INTAKE:

OF 8OZ GLASSES

❑ ❑

❑ ❑

❑ ❑

❑ ❑

❑ ❑

COMMENTS · NOTES · PROGRESS

_____

_____

_____

_____

_____

DATE:_____ WEEK#:_____ DAY#:_____   WEIGHT:_____

Helpful Tips

Daily Workout Journal

Allow two
days of rest
each week
for muscles
being strength
trained.

CARDIOVASCULAR EXERCISE   STRETCHING/WARMUP: yes ☐ no ☐

Time	Exercise Type	Minutes	Distance	Pace/ Setting	Cal. Burned
CARDIO EXERCISE TOTALS:					

COMMENTS:

STRENGTH TRAINING   TARGET AREA: upper body ☐ lower body ☐ abs ☐

Exercise Type	Muscle Group	SET 1 Reps/Wt.	SET 2 Reps/Wt.	SET 3 Reps/Wt.	SET 4 Reps/Wt.
STRENGTH TRAINING TOTALS:					

WORKOUT
REMINDER:

_____

_____

_____

_____

_____

_____

COMMENTS:

OTHER · GROUP EXERCISE   STRETCHING/WARMUP: yes ☐ no ☐

Time	Exercise Type	Minutes	Cal. Burned
OTHER · GROUP EXERCISE TOTALS:			

COMMENTS:

DAILY GOAL(S) _____

_____

_____

DAILY GOALS ACHIEVED

FLEXIBILITY · RELAXATION · MEDITATION

Activity Performed	Minutes
FLEXIBILITY · RELAXATION · MEDITATION TOTALS:	
COMMENTS:	

NUTRITIONAL INTAKE

Food Item	amt.	cal.	fat gms	protein gms	carbs gms	fiber gms
BREAKFAST:						
LUNCH:						
DINNER:						
SNACKS:						
INTAKE TOTALS:						

VITAMINS & SUPPLEMENTS

Type: _____
Qty: _____

Type: _____
Qty: _____

Type: _____
Qty: _____

Type: _____
Qty: _____

WATER INTAKE:

OF 8OZ GLASSES

❑ ❑

❑ ❑

❑ ❑

❑ ❑

❑ ❑

COMMENTS · NOTES · PROGRESS

_____

_____

_____

_____

_____

DATE:_____ WEEK#:_____ DAY#:_____ WEIGHT:_____

ENERGY LEVELS: low ❑ med ❑ high ❑

Daily Workout Journal

The old saying,
"No pain,
no gain" is
false. If you
experience
pain, stop
immediately.
If pain does
not subside,
contact a
medical
professional.

CARDIOVASCULAR EXERCISE   STRETCHING/WARMUP: yes ❑ no ❑

Time	Exercise Type	Minutes	Distance	Pace/ Setting	Cal. Burned
CARDIO EXERCISE TOTALS:					

COMMENTS:

STRENGTH TRAINING   TARGET AREA: upper body ❑ lower body ❑ abs ❑

Exercise Type	Muscle Group	SET 1 Reps/Wt.	SET 2 Reps/Wt.	SET 3 Reps/Wt.	SET 4 Reps/Wt.
STRENGTH TRAINING TOTALS:					

COMMENTS:

OTHER · GROUP EXERCISE   STRETCHING/WARMUP: yes ❑ no ❑

Time	Exercise Type	Minutes	Cal. Burned
OTHER · GROUP EXERCISE TOTALS:			

COMMENTS:

I DID IT!

DAILY GOALS
ACHIEVED

FLEXIBILITY · RELAXATION · MEDITATION

Activity Performed	Minutes
FLEXIBILITY · RELAXATION · MEDITATION TOTALS:	
COMMENTS:	

NUTRITIONAL INTAKE

Food Item	amt.	cal.	fat gms	protein gms	carbs gms	fiber gms
BREAKFAST:						
LUNCH:						
DINNER:						
SNACKS:						
INTAKE TOTALS:						

VITAMINS & SUPPLEMENTS

Type:
Qty:

Type:
Qty:

Type:
Qty:

Type:
Qty:

WATER INTAKE:

OF 8OZ GLASSES

❏ ❏
❏ ❏
❏ ❏
❏ ❏
❏ ❏

COMMENTS · NOTES · PROGRESS

DATE:_____ WEEK#:_____ DAY#:_____   WEIGHT:_____

ENERGY LEVELS: low ❑ med ❑ high ❑

Daily Workout Journal

CARDIOVASCULAR EXERCISE   STRETCHING/WARMUP: yes ❑ no ❑

Time	Exercise Type	Minutes	Distance	Pace/ Setting	Cal. Burned
CARDIO EXERCISE TOTALS:					

COMMENTS:

STRENGTH TRAINING   TARGET AREA: upper body ❑ lower body ❑ abs ❑

Exercise Type	Muscle Group	SET 1 Reps/Wt.	SET 2 Reps/Wt.	SET 3 Reps/Wt.	SET 4 Reps/Wt.
STRENGTH TRAINING TOTALS:					

**WORKOUT
REMINDER:**

_____

_____

_____

_____

_____

COMMENTS:

_____

OTHER · GROUP EXERCISE   STRETCHING/WARMUP: yes ❑ no ❑

_____

Time	Exercise Type	Minutes	Cal. Burned
OTHER · GROUP EXERCISE TOTALS:			

_____

COMMENTS:

_____

DAILY GOAL(S) _____

_____

_____

**DAILY GOALS
ACHIEVED**

FLEXIBILITY · RELAXATION · MEDITATION

Activity Performed	Minutes
FLEXIBILITY · RELAXATION · MEDITATION TOTALS:	
COMMENTS:	

NUTRITIONAL INTAKE

Food Item	amt.	cal.	fat gms	protein gms	carbs gms	fiber gms
BREAKFAST:						
LUNCH:						
DINNER:						
SNACKS:						
INTAKE TOTALS:						

**VITAMINS &
SUPPLEMENTS**

Type: _____

Qty: _____

Type: _____

Qty: _____

Type: _____

Qty: _____

Type: _____

Qty: _____

WATER INTAKE:

OF 8OZ GLASSES

❏ ❏

❏ ❏

❏ ❏

❏ ❏

❏ ❏

COMMENTS · NOTES · PROGRESS

_____

_____

_____

_____

_____

DATE:_____ WEEK#:_____ DAY#:_____ WEIGHT:_____

ENERGY LEVELS: low ☐ med ☐ high ☐

Daily Workout Journal

It takes time
for your brain
to receive the
signal that
your stomach
is full. Eat
slowly so
you don't eat
more than
necessary. If
you've eaten
an entire meal
but still feel
hungry, wait
at least fifteen
minutes
before eating
more.

CARDIOVASCULAR EXERCISE   STRETCHING/WARMUP: yes ☐ no ☐

Time	Exercise Type	Minutes	Distance	Pace/ Setting	Cal. Burned
CARDIO EXERCISE TOTALS:					

COMMENTS:

STRENGTH TRAINING   TARGET AREA: upper body ☐ lower body ☐ abs ☐

Exercise Type	Muscle Group	SET 1 Reps/Wt.	SET 2 Reps/Wt.	SET 3 Reps/Wt.	SET 4 Reps/Wt.
STRENGTH TRAINING TOTALS:					

COMMENTS:

_____

_____

_____

_____

_____

_____

_____

_____

OTHER · GROUP EXERCISE   STRETCHING/WARMUP: yes ☐ no ☐

Time	Exercise Type	Minutes	Cal. Burned
OTHER · GROUP EXERCISE TOTALS:			

COMMENTS:

DAILY GOAL(S) _____

_____

_____

DAILY GOALS
ACHIEVED

FLEXIBILITY · RELAXATION · MEDITATION

Activity Performed	Minutes
FLEXIBILITY · RELAXATION · MEDITATION TOTALS:	
COMMENTS:	

NUTRITIONAL INTAKE

Food Item	amt.	cal.	fat gms	protein gms	carbs gms	fiber gms
BREAKFAST:						
LUNCH:						
DINNER:						
SNACKS:						
INTAKE TOTALS:						

VITAMINS & SUPPLEMENTS

Type: _____

Qty: _____

Type: _____

Qty: _____

Type: _____

Qty: _____

Type: _____

Qty: _____

WATER INTAKE:

OF 8OZ GLASSES

❑ ❑

❑ ❑

❑ ❑

❑ ❑

❑ ❑

COMMENTS · NOTES · PROGRESS

_____

_____

_____

_____

_____

DATE:_____ WEEK#:_____ DAY#:_____   WEIGHT:_____

ENERGY LEVELS: low ❑ med ❑ high ❑

Daily Workout Journal

CARDIOVASCULAR EXERCISE   STRETCHING/WARMUP: yes ❑ no ❑

Time	Exercise Type	Minutes	Distance	Pace/ Setting	Cal. Burned
CARDIO EXERCISE TOTALS:					

COMMENTS:

STRENGTH TRAINING   TARGET AREA: upper body ❑ lower body ❑ abs ❑

Exercise Type	Muscle Group	SET 1 Reps/Wt.	SET 2 Reps/Wt.	SET 3 Reps/Wt.	SET 4 Reps/Wt.
STRENGTH TRAINING TOTALS:					

WORKOUT REMINDER:

_____

_____

_____

_____

_____

COMMENTS:

OTHER · GROUP EXERCISE   STRETCHING/WARMUP: yes ❑ no ❑

Time	Exercise Type	Minutes	Cal. Burned
OTHER · GROUP EXERCISE TOTALS:			

COMMENTS:

FLEXIBILITY · RELAXATION · MEDITATION

Activity Performed	Minutes
FLEXIBILITY · RELAXATION · MEDITATION TOTALS:	
COMMENTS:	

NUTRITIONAL INTAKE

Food Item	amt.	cal.	fat gms	protein gms	carbs gms	fiber gms
BREAKFAST:						
LUNCH:						
DINNER:						
SNACKS:						
INTAKE TOTALS:						

VITAMINS & SUPPLEMENTS

Type: _____
Qty: _____

Type: _____
Qty: _____

Type: _____
Qty: _____

Type: _____
Qty: _____

WATER INTAKE:
OF 8oz GLASSES

❑ ❑
❑ ❑
❑ ❑
❑ ❑
❑ ❑

COMMENTS · NOTES · PROGRESS

DATE:_____ WEEK#:_____ DAY#:_____   WEIGHT:_____

ENERGY LEVELS: low ❑ med ❑ high ❑

Daily Workout Journal

It is
important to
vary the types
of vegetables
you eat.
Different
vegetables
contain
different
nutrients.

CARDIOVASCULAR EXERCISE STRETCHING/WARMUP: yes ❑ no ❑

Time	Exercise Type	Minutes	Distance	Pace/ Setting	Cal. Burned
CARDIO EXERCISE TOTALS:					

COMMENTS:

STRENGTH TRAINING TARGET AREA: upper body ❑ lower body ❑ abs ❑

Exercise Type	Muscle Group	SET 1 Reps/Wt.	SET 2 Reps/Wt.	SET 3 Reps/Wt.	SET 4 Reps/Wt.
STRENGTH TRAINING TOTALS:					

WORKOUT
REMINDER:

_____

_____

_____

_____

COMMENTS:

_____

_____

_____

OTHER · GROUP EXERCISE STRETCHING/WARMUP: yes ❑ no ❑

Time	Exercise Type	Minutes	Cal. Burned
OTHER · GROUP EXERCISE TOTALS:			

COMMENTS:

DAILY GOAL(S) _____

_____

_____

**DAILY GOALS
ACHIEVED**

FLEXIBILITY · RELAXATION · MEDITATION

Activity Performed	Minutes
FLEXIBILITY · RELAXATION · MEDITATION TOTALS:	
COMMENTS:	

NUTRITIONAL INTAKE

Food Item	amt.	cal.	fat gms	protein gms	carbs gms	fiber gms
BREAKFAST:						
LUNCH:						
DINNER:						
SNACKS:						
INTAKE TOTALS:						

**VITAMINS &
SUPPLEMENTS**

Type: _____

Qty: _____

Type: _____

Qty: _____

Type: _____

Qty: _____

Type: _____

Qty: _____

WATER INTAKE:

OF 8OZ GLASSES

❑ ❑

❑ ❑

❑ ❑

❑ ❑

❑ ❑

COMMENTS · NOTES · PROGRESS

_____

_____

_____

_____

_____

ENERGY LEVELS: low ☐ med ☐ high ☐

Helpful Tips

Daily Workout Journal

Varying
your fitness
activities
will help
you combat
boredom.

CARDIOVASCULAR EXERCISE   STRETCHING/WARMUP: yes ☐ no ☐

Time	Exercise Type	Minutes	Distance	Pace/ Setting	Cal. Burned
CARDIO EXERCISE TOTALS:					

COMMENTS:

STRENGTH TRAINING   TARGET AREA: upper body ☐ lower body ☐ abs ☐

Exercise Type	Muscle Group	SET 1 Reps/Wt.	SET 2 Reps/Wt.	SET 3 Reps/Wt.	SET 4 Reps/Wt.
STRENGTH TRAINING TOTALS:					

WORKOUT REMINDER:

_____

_____

_____

_____

_____

COMMENTS:

OTHER · GROUP EXERCISE   STRETCHING/WARMUP: yes ☐ no ☐

Time	Exercise Type	Minutes	Cal. Burned
OTHER · GROUP EXERCISE TOTALS:			

_____

_____

_____

_____

COMMENTS:

DAILY GOAL(S) _____

_____

_____

**DAILY GOALS
ACHIEVED**

FLEXIBILITY · RELAXATION · MEDITATION

Activity Performed	Minutes
FLEXIBILITY · RELAXATION · MEDITATION TOTALS:	
COMMENTS:	

NUTRITIONAL INTAKE

Food Item	amt.	cal.	fat gms	protein gms	carbs gms	fiber gms
BREAKFAST:						
LUNCH:						
DINNER:						
SNACKS:						
INTAKE TOTALS:						

**VITAMINS &
SUPPLEMENTS**

Type: _____

Qty: _____

Type: _____

Qty: _____

Type: _____

Qty: _____

Type: _____

Qty: _____

WATER INTAKE:

OF 8OZ GLASSES

❏ ❏

❏ ❏

❏ ❏

❏ ❏

❏ ❏

COMMENTS · NOTES · PROGRESS

_____

_____

_____

_____

_____

DATE:_____ WEEK#:_____ DAY#:_____ WEIGHT:_____

ENERGY LEVELS: low ☐ med ☐ high ☐

Daily Workout Journal

Studies show
that drinking
green tea in
moderation
can benefit
your health.
Green tea
contains anti-
oxidants,
lowers LDL
("bad")
cholesterol,
stimulates
your
metabolism
and boosts
your immune
system.

CARDIOVASCULAR EXERCISE   STRETCHING/WARMUP: yes ☐ no ☐

Time	Exercise Type	Minutes	Distance	Pace/ Setting	Cal. Burned
CARDIO EXERCISE TOTALS:					

COMMENTS:

STRENGTH TRAINING   TARGET AREA: upper body ☐ lower body ☐ abs ☐

Exercise Type	Muscle Group	SET 1 Reps/Wt.	SET 2 Reps/Wt.	SET 3 Reps/Wt.	SET 4 Reps/Wt.
STRENGTH TRAINING TOTALS:					

COMMENTS:

OTHER · GROUP EXERCISE   STRETCHING/WARMUP: yes ☐ no ☐

Time	Exercise Type	Minutes	Cal. Burned
OTHER · GROUP EXERCISE TOTALS:			

COMMENTS:

DAILY GOAL(S) _____

_____

_____

**DAILY GOALS
ACHIEVED**

FLEXIBILITY · RELAXATION · MEDITATION

Activity Performed	Minutes
FLEXIBILITY · RELAXATION · MEDITATION TOTALS:	
COMMENTS:	

NUTRITIONAL INTAKE

Food Item	amt.	cal.	fat gms	protein gms	carbs gms	fiber gms
BREAKFAST:						
LUNCH:						
DINNER:						
SNACKS:						
INTAKE TOTALS:						

VITAMINS & SUPPLEMENTS

Type: _____

Qty: _____

Type: _____

Qty: _____

Type: _____

Qty: _____

Type: _____

Qty: _____

WATER INTAKE:

OF 8OZ GLASSES

❑ ❑

❑ ❑

❑ ❑

❑ ❑

❑ ❑

COMMENTS · NOTES · PROGRESS

_____

_____

_____

_____

_____

_____

ENERGY LEVELS: low ❑ med ❑ high ❑

Daily Workout Journal

Helpful Tips

Working out first thing in the morning boosts your metabolism for the whole day, encouraging weight loss, even during periods of inactivity.

CARDIOVASCULAR EXERCISE   STRETCHING/WARMUP: yes ❑ no ❑

Time	Exercise Type	Minutes	Distance	Pace/Setting	Cal. Burned
CARDIO EXERCISE TOTALS:					

COMMENTS:

STRENGTH TRAINING   TARGET AREA: upper body ❑ lower body ❑ abs ❑

Exercise Type	Muscle Group	SET 1 Reps/Wt.	SET 2 Reps/Wt.	SET 3 Reps/Wt.	SET 4 Reps/Wt.
STRENGTH TRAINING TOTALS:					

WORKOUT REMINDER:

_____

_____

_____

_____

_____

COMMENTS:

OTHER · GROUP EXERCISE   STRETCHING/WARMUP: yes ❑ no ❑

Time	Exercise Type	Minutes	Cal. Burned
OTHER · GROUP EXERCISE TOTALS:			

COMMENTS:

DAILY GOAL(S)

I DID IT!

DAILY GOALS ACHIEVED

FLEXIBILITY · RELAXATION · MEDITATION

Activity Performed	Minutes
FLEXIBILITY · RELAXATION · MEDITATION TOTALS:	
COMMENTS:	

NUTRITIONAL INTAKE

Food Item	amt.	cal.	fat gms	protein gms	carbs gms	fiber gms
BREAKFAST:						
LUNCH:						
DINNER:						
SNACKS:						
INTAKE TOTALS:						

VITAMINS & SUPPLEMENTS

Type:

Qty:

Type:

Qty:

Type:

Qty:

Type:

Qty:

WATER INTAKE:

OF 8oz GLASSES

❏ ❏
❏ ❏
❏ ❏
❏ ❏
❏ ❏

COMMENTS · NOTES · PROGRESS

DATE:_____ WEEK#:_____ DAY#:_____   WEIGHT:_____

ENERGY LEVELS: low ☐ med ☐ high ☐

Daily Workout Journal

A "do-or-die"
attitude will
set you up
for failure.
Plan for
setbacks and
concentrate
on long-term
progress.

CARDIOVASCULAR EXERCISE   STRETCHING/WARMUP: yes ☐ no ☐

Time	Exercise Type	Minutes	Distance	Pace/Setting	Cal. Burned
CARDIO EXERCISE TOTALS:					

COMMENTS:

STRENGTH TRAINING   TARGET AREA: upper body ☐ lower body ☐ abs ☐

Exercise Type	Muscle Group	SET 1 Reps/Wt.	SET 2 Reps/Wt.	SET 3 Reps/Wt.	SET 4 Reps/Wt.
STRENGTH TRAINING TOTALS:					

COMMENTS:

OTHER · GROUP EXERCISE   STRETCHING/WARMUP: yes ☐ no ☐

Time	Exercise Type	Minutes	Cal. Burned
OTHER · GROUP EXERCISE TOTALS:			

COMMENTS:

**DAILY GOALS
ACHIEVED**

FLEXIBILITY · RELAXATION · MEDITATION

Activity Performed	Minutes
FLEXIBILITY · RELAXATION · MEDITATION TOTALS:	
COMMENTS:	

NUTRITIONAL INTAKE

Food Item	amt.	cal.	fat gms	protein gms	carbs gms	fiber gms
BREAKFAST:						
LUNCH:						
DINNER:						
SNACKS:						
INTAKE TOTALS:						

**VITAMINS &
SUPPLEMENTS**

Type:
Qty:

Type:
Qty:

Type:
Qty:

Type:
Qty:

WATER INTAKE:
OF 8oz GLASSES

❏ ❏
❏ ❏
❏ ❏
❏ ❏
❏ ❏

COMMENTS · NOTES · PROGRESS

DATE:_____ WEEK#:_____ DAY#:_____ WEIGHT:_____

ENERGY LEVELS: low ☐ med ☐ high ☐

Daily Workout Journal

Be honest
with yourself.
If you cheat
on your
diet or
overindulge,
admit to
having
done that
and resume
your diet.
Kidding
yourself
and making
excuses will
only keep you
from reaching
your goals.

CARDIOVASCULAR EXERCISE   STRETCHING/WARMUP: yes ☐ no ☐

Time	Exercise Type	Minutes	Distance	Pace/ Setting	Cal. Burned
CARDIO EXERCISE TOTALS:					

COMMENTS:

STRENGTH TRAINING   TARGET AREA: upper body ☐ lower body ☐ abs ☐

Exercise Type	Muscle Group	SET 1 Reps/Wt.	SET 2 Reps/Wt.	SET 3 Reps/Wt.	SET 4 Reps/Wt.
STRENGTH TRAINING TOTALS:					

COMMENTS:

OTHER · GROUP EXERCISE   STRETCHING/WARMUP: yes ☐ no ☐

Time	Exercise Type	Minutes	Cal. Burned
OTHER · GROUP EXERCISE TOTALS:			

COMMENTS:

FLEXIBILITY · RELAXATION · MEDITATION

Activity Performed	Minutes
FLEXIBILITY · RELAXATION · MEDITATION TOTALS:	

COMMENTS:

NUTRITIONAL INTAKE

Food Item	amt.	cal.	fat gms	protein gms	carbs gms	fiber gms
BREAKFAST:						
LUNCH:						
DINNER:						
SNACKS:						
INTAKE TOTALS:						

VITAMINS & SUPPLEMENTS

Type: _____
Qty: _____

Type: _____
Qty: _____

Type: _____
Qty: _____

Type: _____
Qty: _____

WATER INTAKE:

OF 8OZ GLASSES

❑ ❑
❑ ❑
❑ ❑
❑ ❑
❑ ❑

COMMENTS · NOTES · PROGRESS

DATE:_____ WEEK#:_____ DAY#:_____ WEIGHT:_____

ENERGY LEVELS: low ☐ med ☐ high ☐

Daily Workout Journal

Getting fit
can transform
your life. The
increased
confidence
and self-
esteem you
experience
may enhance
your
enjoyment
of both your
professional
and social
life.

CARDIOVASCULAR EXERCISE   STRETCHING/WARMUP: yes ☐ no ☐

Time	Exercise Type	Minutes	Distance	Pace/ Setting	Cal. Burned
CARDIO EXERCISE TOTALS:					

COMMENTS:

STRENGTH TRAINING   TARGET AREA: upper body ☐ lower body ☐ abs ☐

Exercise Type	Muscle Group	SET 1 Reps/Wt.	SET 2 Reps/Wt.	SET 3 Reps/Wt.	SET 4 Reps/Wt.
STRENGTH TRAINING TOTALS:					

WORKOUT
REMINDER:

_____
_____
_____
_____
_____
_____
_____
_____
_____
_____
_____

COMMENTS:

OTHER·GROUP EXERCISE   STRETCHING/WARMUP: yes ☐ no ☐

Time	Exercise Type	Minutes	Cal. Burned
OTHER·GROUP EXERCISE TOTALS:			

COMMENTS:

DAILY GOAL(S) _____

**DAILY GOALS
ACHIEVED**

FLEXIBILITY · RELAXATION · MEDITATION

Activity Performed	Minutes
FLEXIBILITY · RELAXATION · MEDITATION TOTALS:	
COMMENTS:	

NUTRITIONAL INTAKE

Food Item	amt.	cal.	fat gms	protein gms	carbs gms	fiber gms
BREAKFAST:						
LUNCH:						
DINNER:						
SNACKS:						
INTAKE TOTALS:						

VITAMINS & SUPPLEMENTS

Type: _____
Qty: _____

Type: _____
Qty: _____

Type: _____
Qty: _____

Type: _____
Qty: _____

WATER INTAKE:
OF 8OZ GLASSES

☐ ☐
☐ ☐
☐ ☐
☐ ☐
☐ ☐

COMMENTS · NOTES · PROGRESS

_____

_____

_____

_____

_____

DATE:_____ WEEK#:_____ DAY#:_____ WEIGHT:_____

ENERGY LEVELS: low ☐ med ☐ high ☐

Daily Workout Journal

You can
save money
by using
an Internet
personal
trainer,
someone
who will help
you select
appropriate
exercise
routines and
help you
track your
results via
e-mail. If
you decide
to work with
an Internet
trainer, be
certain to
find one who
is educated
and certified.

CARDIOVASCULAR EXERCISE   STRETCHING/WARMUP: yes ☐ no ☐

Time	Exercise Type	Minutes	Distance	Pace/Setting	Cal. Burned
CARDIO EXERCISE TOTALS:					

COMMENTS:

STRENGTH TRAINING   TARGET AREA: upper body ☐ lower body ☐ abs ☐

Exercise Type	Muscle Group	SET 1 Reps/Wt.	SET 2 Reps/Wt.	SET 3 Reps/Wt.	SET 4 Reps/Wt.
STRENGTH TRAINING TOTALS:					

COMMENTS:

OTHER·GROUP EXERCISE   STRETCHING/WARMUP: yes ☐ no ☐

Time	Exercise Type	Minutes	Cal. Burned
OTHER·GROUP EXERCISE TOTALS:			

COMMENTS:

FLEXIBILITY · RELAXATION · MEDITATION

Activity Performed	Minutes
FLEXIBILITY · RELAXATION · MEDITATION TOTALS:	

COMMENTS:

NUTRITIONAL INTAKE

Food Item	amt.	cal.	fat gms	protein gms	carbs gms	fiber gms
BREAKFAST:						
LUNCH:						
DINNER:						
SNACKS:						
INTAKE TOTALS:						

VITAMINS & SUPPLEMENTS

Type: _____
Qty: _____

Type: _____
Qty: _____

Type: _____
Qty: _____

Type: _____
Qty: _____

WATER INTAKE:
OF 8OZ GLASSES

❑ ❑
❑ ❑
❑ ❑
❑ ❑
❑ ❑

COMMENTS · NOTES · PROGRESS

_____
_____
_____
_____
_____
_____

DATE:_____ WEEK#:_____ DAY#:_____   WEIGHT:_____

ENERGY LEVELS: low ☐ med ☐ high ☐

Helpful Tips

Daily Workout Journal

It is important
to celebrate
your
successes.
Indulge in
a favorite
activity or
purchase a
new outfit
to celebrate
reaching your
fitness goals.

CARDIOVASCULAR EXERCISE   STRETCHING/WARMUP: yes ☐ no ☐

Time	Exercise Type	Minutes	Distance	Pace/Setting	Cal. Burned
CARDIO EXERCISE TOTALS:					

COMMENTS:

STRENGTH TRAINING   TARGET AREA: upper body ☐ lower body ☐ abs ☐

Exercise Type	Muscle Group	SET 1 Reps/Wt.	SET 2 Reps/Wt.	SET 3 Reps/Wt.	SET 4 Reps/Wt.
STRENGTH TRAINING TOTALS:					

**WORKOUT
REMINDER:**

COMMENTS:

OTHER · GROUP EXERCISE   STRETCHING/WARMUP: yes ☐ no ☐

Time	Exercise Type	Minutes	Cal. Burned
OTHER · GROUP EXERCISE TOTALS:			

COMMENTS:

DAILY GOAL(S) _____

_____

_____

DAILY GOALS
ACHIEVED

FLEXIBILITY · RELAXATION · MEDITATION

Activity Performed	Minutes
FLEXIBILITY · RELAXATION · MEDITATION TOTALS:	
COMMENTS:	

NUTRITIONAL INTAKE

Food Item	amt.	cal.	fat gms	protein gms	carbs gms	fiber gms
BREAKFAST:						
LUNCH:						
DINNER:						
SNACKS:						
INTAKE TOTALS:						

VITAMINS & SUPPLEMENTS

Type: _____
Qty: _____

Type: _____
Qty: _____

Type: _____
Qty: _____

Type: _____
Qty: _____

WATER INTAKE:
OF 8OZ GLASSES

❏ ❏

❏ ❏

❏ ❏

❏ ❏

❏ ❏

COMMENTS · NOTES · PROGRESS

_____

_____

_____

_____

_____

DATE:_____ WEEK#:_____ DAY#:_____   WEIGHT:_____

Helpful Tips

Daily Workout Journal

Recent studies have shown that regular physical activity can help women manage the symptoms of menopause. Women who maintain a regular fitness routine experience a decrease in the anxiety and depression that often accompanies menopause.

CARDIOVASCULAR EXERCISE   STRETCHING/WARMUP: yes ☐ no ☐

Time	Exercise Type	Minutes	Distance	Pace/ Setting	Cal. Burned
CARDIO EXERCISE TOTALS:					

COMMENTS:

STRENGTH TRAINING   TARGET AREA: upper body ☐ lower body ☐ abs ☐

Exercise Type	Muscle Group	SET 1 Reps/Wt.	SET 2 Reps/Wt.	SET 3 Reps/Wt.	SET 4 Reps/Wt.
STRENGTH TRAINING TOTALS:					

WORKOUT REMINDER:

_____

_____

_____

COMMENTS:

OTHER · GROUP EXERCISE   STRETCHING/WARMUP: yes ☐ no ☐

Time	Exercise Type	Minutes	Cal. Burned
OTHER · GROUP EXERCISE TOTALS:			

COMMENTS:

**DAILY GOALS
ACHIEVED**

FLEXIBILITY · RELAXATION · MEDITATION

Activity Performed	Minutes
FLEXIBILITY · RELAXATION · MEDITATION TOTALS:	

COMMENTS:

NUTRITIONAL INTAKE

Food Item	amt.	cal.	fat gms	protein gms	carbs gms	fiber gms
BREAKFAST:						
LUNCH:						
DINNER:						
SNACKS:						
INTAKE TOTALS:						

VITAMINS & SUPPLEMENTS

Type:
Qty:

Type:
Qty:

Type:
Qty:

Type:
Qty:

WATER INTAKE:
OF 8OZ GLASSES

❑ ❑
❑ ❑
❑ ❑
❑ ❑
❑ ❑

COMMENTS · NOTES · PROGRESS

DATE:_____ WEEK#:_____ DAY#:_____   WEIGHT:_____

Helpful Tips

Daily Workout Journal

CARDIOVASCULAR EXERCISE   STRETCHING/WARMUP: yes ☐ no ☐

Working out offers many physical and emotional benefits to pregnant women. Exercise may help prevent excessive weight gain, swelling of your hands and feet, leg cramps, varicose veins, insomnia, fatigue and constipation. If you are pregnant it is extremely important to contact your doctor before beginning any fitness routine.

Time	Exercise Type	Minutes	Distance	Pace/Setting	Cal. Burned
CARDIO EXERCISE TOTALS:					

COMMENTS:

STRENGTH TRAINING   TARGET AREA: upper body ☐   lower body ☐   abs ☐

Exercise Type	Muscle Group	SET 1 Reps/Wt.	SET 2 Reps/Wt.	SET 3 Reps/Wt.	SET 4 Reps/Wt.
STRENGTH TRAINING TOTALS:					

WORKOUT REMINDER:

COMMENTS:

OTHER·GROUP EXERCISE   STRETCHING/WARMUP: yes ☐ no ☐

Time	Exercise Type	Minutes	Cal. Burned
OTHER·GROUP EXERCISE TOTALS:			

COMMENTS:

DAILY GOAL(S) _____

DAILY GOALS
ACHIEVED

FLEXIBILITY · RELAXATION · MEDITATION

Activity Performed	Minutes
FLEXIBILITY · RELAXATION · MEDITATION TOTALS:	
COMMENTS:	

NUTRITIONAL INTAKE

Food Item	amt.	cal.	fat gms	protein gms	carbs gms	fiber gms
BREAKFAST:						
LUNCH:						
DINNER:						
SNACKS:						
INTAKE TOTALS:						

VITAMINS & SUPPLEMENTS

Type: _____
Qty: _____

Type: _____
Qty: _____

Type: _____
Qty: _____

Type: _____
Qty: _____

WATER INTAKE:

OF 8OZ GLASSES

❑ ❑
❑ ❑
❑ ❑
❑ ❑
❑ ❑

COMMENTS · NOTES · PROGRESS

_____

_____

_____

_____

_____

DATE:_____ WEEK#:_____ DAY#:_____ WEIGHT:_____

ENERGY LEVELS: low ❑ med ❑ high ❑

Helpful Tips

Daily Workout Journal

Exercise can decrease your risk of developing Type-2 diabetes.

CARDIOVASCULAR EXERCISE   STRETCHING/WARMUP: yes ❑ no ❑

Time	Exercise Type	Minutes	Distance	Pace/ Setting	Cal. Burned

CARDIO EXERCISE TOTALS:

COMMENTS:

STRENGTH TRAINING   TARGET AREA: upper body ❑ lower body ❑ abs ❑

Exercise Type	Muscle Group	SET 1 Reps/Wt.	SET 2 Reps/Wt.	SET 3 Reps/Wt.	SET 4 Reps/Wt.

STRENGTH TRAINING TOTALS:

COMMENTS:

WORKOUT REMINDER:

OTHER · GROUP EXERCISE   STRETCHING/WARMUP: yes ❑ no ❑

Time	Exercise Type	Minutes	Cal. Burned

OTHER · GROUP EXERCISE TOTALS:

COMMENTS:

DAILY GOAL(S) _____

_____

FLEXIBILITY · RELAXATION · MEDITATION

Activity Performed	Minutes
FLEXIBILITY · RELAXATION · MEDITATION TOTALS:	
COMMENTS:	

NUTRITIONAL INTAKE

Food Item	amt.	cal.	fat gms	protein gms	carbs gms	fiber gms
BREAKFAST:						
LUNCH:						
DINNER:						
SNACKS:						
INTAKE TOTALS:						

VITAMINS & SUPPLEMENTS

Type: _____
Qty: _____

Type: _____
Qty: _____

Type: _____
Qty: _____

Type: _____
Qty: _____

WATER INTAKE:
OF 8OZ GLASSES

❑ ❑

❑ ❑

❑ ❑

❑ ❑

❑ ❑

COMMENTS · NOTES · PROGRESS

_____

_____

_____

_____

_____

DATE:_____ WEEK#:_____ DAY#:_____ WEIGHT:_____

Helpful Tips

Daily Workout Journal

Research
shows
that those
suffering from
asthma may
benefit from
a regular
exercise
routine.
Studies have
shown that
a tolerance
for physical
exertion
can be built
up slowly
over time.
If you have
asthma, it is
important
that you
talk to your
doctor before
beginning
any fitness
routine.

**WORKOUT
REMINDER:**

_____

_____

_____

_____

_____

_____

_____

_____

_____

_____

CARDIOVASCULAR EXERCISE   STRETCHING/WARMUP: yes ❑ no ❑

Time	Exercise Type	Minutes	Distance	Pace/ Setting	Cal. Burned
CARDIO EXERCISE TOTALS:					

COMMENTS:

STRENGTH TRAINING   TARGET AREA: upper body ❑ lower body ❑ abs ❑

Exercise Type	Muscle Group	SET 1 Reps/Wt.	SET 2 Reps/Wt.	SET 3 Reps/Wt.	SET 4 Reps/Wt.
STRENGTH TRAINING TOTALS:					

COMMENTS:

OTHER · GROUP EXERCISE   STRETCHING/WARMUP: yes ❑ no ❑

Time	Exercise Type	Minutes	Cal. Burned
OTHER · GROUP EXERCISE TOTALS:			

COMMENTS:

DAILY GOALS ACHIEVED

FLEXIBILITY · RELAXATION · MEDITATION

Activity Performed	Minutes
FLEXIBILITY · RELAXATION · MEDITATION TOTALS:	
COMMENTS:	

NUTRITIONAL INTAKE

Food Item	amt.	cal.	fat gms	protein gms	carbs gms	fiber gms
BREAKFAST:						
LUNCH:						
DINNER:						
SNACKS:						
INTAKE TOTALS:						

VITAMINS & SUPPLEMENTS

Type: _____
Qty: _____

Type: _____
Qty: _____

Type: _____
Qty: _____

Type: _____
Qty: _____

WATER INTAKE:

OF 8OZ GLASSES

❑ ❑
❑ ❑
❑ ❑
❑ ❑
❑ ❑

COMMENTS · NOTES · PROGRESS

_____

_____

_____

_____

_____

_____

DATE:_____ WEEK#:_____ DAY#:_____   WEIGHT:_____

Helpful Tips

Daily Workout Journal

If you usually
work out
indoors, add
an outside
activity, such
as hiking or
bicycle riding,
to get some
fresh air
during your
workout.

CARDIOVASCULAR EXERCISE   STRETCHING/WARMUP: yes ☐ no ☐

Time	Exercise Type	Minutes	Distance	Pace/ Setting	Cal. Burned
CARDIO EXERCISE TOTALS:					

COMMENTS:

STRENGTH TRAINING   TARGET AREA: upper body ☐ lower body ☐ abs ☐

Exercise Type	Muscle Group	SET 1 Reps/Wt.	SET 2 Reps/Wt.	SET 3 Reps/Wt.	SET 4 Reps/Wt.
STRENGTH TRAINING TOTALS:					

WORKOUT REMINDER:

_____

_____

_____

_____

_____

_____

_____

_____

_____

COMMENTS:

OTHER · GROUP EXERCISE   STRETCHING/WARMUP: yes ☐ no ☐

Time	Exercise Type	Minutes	Cal. Burned
OTHER · GROUP EXERCISE TOTALS:			

COMMENTS:

DAILY GOAL(S) _____

_____

_____

**DAILY GOALS
ACHIEVED**

FLEXIBILITY · RELAXATION · MEDITATION

Activity Performed	Minutes
FLEXIBILITY · RELAXATION · MEDITATION TOTALS:	
COMMENTS:	

NUTRITIONAL INTAKE

Food Item	amt.	cal.	fat gms	protein gms	carbs gms	fiber gms
BREAKFAST:						
LUNCH:						
DINNER:						
SNACKS:						
INTAKE TOTALS:						

**VITAMINS &
SUPPLEMENTS**

Type: _____

Qty: _____

Type: _____

Qty: _____

Type: _____

Qty: _____

Type: _____

Qty: _____

WATER INTAKE:

OF 8OZ GLASSES

❑ ❑

❑ ❑

❑ ❑

❑ ❑

❑ ❑

COMMENTS · NOTES · PROGRESS

_____

_____

_____

_____

_____

DATE:_____ WEEK#:_____ DAY#:_____ WEIGHT:_____

Helpful Tips

Daily Workout Journal

Research shows that those who regularly exercise are less likely to get sick. During moderate exercise, white blood cells and other immunity boosting cells circulate through the body more quickly. This increased circulation allows these cells to kill bacteria and viruses more efficiently.

CARDIOVASCULAR EXERCISE   STRETCHING/WARMUP: yes ☐ no ☐

Time	Exercise Type	Minutes	Distance	Pace/ Setting	Cal. Burned
CARDIO EXERCISE TOTALS:					

COMMENTS:

STRENGTH TRAINING   TARGET AREA: upper body ☐ lower body ☐ abs ☐

Exercise Type	Muscle Group	SET 1 Reps/Wt.	SET 2 Reps/Wt.	SET 3 Reps/Wt.	SET 4 Reps/Wt.
STRENGTH TRAINING TOTALS:					

COMMENTS:

WORKOUT REMINDER:

_____

_____

_____

_____

_____

_____

_____

OTHER · GROUP EXERCISE   STRETCHING/WARMUP: yes ☐ no ☐

Time	Exercise Type	Minutes	Cal. Burned
OTHER · GROUP EXERCISE TOTALS:			

COMMENTS:

DAILY GOAL(S) _____

_____

_____

**DAILY GOALS
ACHIEVED**

FLEXIBILITY · RELAXATION · MEDITATION

Activity Performed	Minutes
FLEXIBILITY · RELAXATION · MEDITATION TOTALS:	

COMMENTS:

NUTRITIONAL INTAKE

Food Item	amt.	cal.	fat gms	protein gms	carbs gms	fiber gms
BREAKFAST:						
LUNCH:						
DINNER:						
SNACKS:						
INTAKE TOTALS:						

VITAMINS & SUPPLEMENTS

Type: _____
Qty: _____

Type: _____
Qty: _____

Type: _____
Qty: _____

WATER INTAKE:

OF 8OZ GLASSES

❑ ❑
❑ ❑
❑ ❑
❑ ❑
❑ ❑

COMMENTS · NOTES · PROGRESS

_____

_____

_____

_____

_____

DATE:_____ WEEK#:_____ DAY#:_____ WEIGHT:_____

Helpful Tips

Daily Workout Journal

Avoid New Year's resolution backlash by starting a fitness routine before the holidays.

CARDIOVASCULAR EXERCISE STRETCHING/WARMUP: yes ☐ no ☐

Time	Exercise Type	Minutes	Distance	Pace/Setting	Cal. Burned
CARDIO EXERCISE TOTALS:					

COMMENTS:

STRENGTH TRAINING TARGET AREA: upper body ☐ lower body ☐ abs ☐

Exercise Type	Muscle Group	SET 1 Reps/Wt.	SET 2 Reps/Wt.	SET 3 Reps/Wt.	SET 4 Reps/Wt.
STRENGTH TRAINING TOTALS:					

WORKOUT REMINDER:

_____

_____

_____

_____

_____

COMMENTS:

_____

_____

OTHER · GROUP EXERCISE STRETCHING/WARMUP: yes ☐ no ☐

_____

Time	Exercise Type	Minutes	Cal. Burned
OTHER · GROUP EXERCISE TOTALS:			

COMMENTS:

DAILY GOAL(S) _____

_____

_____

DAILY GOALS
ACHIEVED

FLEXIBILITY · RELAXATION · MEDITATION

Activity Performed	Minutes
FLEXIBILITY · RELAXATION · MEDITATION TOTALS:	
COMMENTS:	

NUTRITIONAL INTAKE

Food Item	amt.	cal.	fat gms	protein gms	carbs gms	fiber gms
BREAKFAST:						
LUNCH:						
DINNER:						
SNACKS:						
INTAKE TOTALS:						

VITAMINS &
SUPPLEMENTS

Type: _____

Qty: _____

Type: _____

Qty: _____

Type: _____

Qty: _____

Type: _____

Qty: _____

WATER INTAKE:

OF 8OZ GLASSES

☐ ☐

☐ ☐

☐ ☐

☐ ☐

☐ ☐

COMMENTS · NOTES · PROGRESS

_____

_____

_____

_____

_____

DATE:_____ WEEK#:_____ DAY#:_____   WEIGHT:_____

Helpful Tips

Daily Workout Journal

Be sure to
use sunscreen
if exercising
outside.

CARDIOVASCULAR EXERCISE   STRETCHING/WARMUP: yes ☐ no ☐

Time	Exercise Type	Minutes	Distance	Pace/ Setting	Cal. Burned
CARDIO EXERCISE TOTALS:					

COMMENTS:

STRENGTH TRAINING   TARGET AREA: upper body ☐ lower body ☐ abs ☐

Exercise Type	Muscle Group	SET 1 Reps/Wt.	SET 2 Reps/Wt.	SET 3 Reps/Wt.	SET 4 Reps/Wt.
STRENGTH TRAINING TOTALS:					

COMMENTS:

WORKOUT REMINDER:

OTHER · GROUP EXERCISE   STRETCHING/WARMUP: yes ☐ no ☐

Time	Exercise Type	Minutes	Cal. Burned
OTHER · GROUP EXERCISE TOTALS:			

COMMENTS:

DAILY GOAL(S)_____

**DAILY GOALS
ACHIEVED**

FLEXIBILITY · RELAXATION · MEDITATION

Activity Performed	Minutes
FLEXIBILITY · RELAXATION · MEDITATION TOTALS:	
COMMENTS:	

NUTRITIONAL INTAKE

Food Item	amt.	cal.	fat gms	protein gms	carbs gms	fiber gms
BREAKFAST:						
LUNCH:						
DINNER:						
SNACKS:						
INTAKE TOTALS:						

VITAMINS & SUPPLEMENTS

Type:_____
Qty:_____

Type:_____
Qty:_____

Type:_____
Qty:_____

Type:_____
Qty:_____

WATER INTAKE:
OF 8OZ GLASSES

❏ ❏
❏ ❏
❏ ❏
❏ ❏
❏ ❏

COMMENTS · NOTES · PROGRESS

DATE:_____ WEEK#:_____ DAY#:_____   WEIGHT:_____

ENERGY LEVELS: low ☐ med ☐ high ☐

Daily Workout Journal

Walking at
a brisk pace
for more than
three hours
a week can
reduce your
risk for heart
disease by up
to 65 percent.

CARDIOVASCULAR EXERCISE STRETCHING/WARMUP: yes ☐ no ☐

Time	Exercise Type	Minutes	Distance	Pace/Setting	Cal. Burned
CARDIO EXERCISE TOTALS:					

COMMENTS:

STRENGTH TRAINING TARGET AREA: upper body ☐ lower body ☐ abs ☐

Exercise Type	Muscle Group	SET 1 Reps/Wt.	SET 2 Reps/Wt.	SET 3 Reps/Wt.	SET 4 Reps/Wt.
STRENGTH TRAINING TOTALS:					

WORKOUT
REMINDER:

_____

_____

_____

_____

COMMENTS:

OTHER · GROUP EXERCISE STRETCHING/WARMUP: yes ☐ no ☐

Time	Exercise Type	Minutes	Cal. Burned
OTHER · GROUP EXERCISE TOTALS:			

COMMENTS:

DAILY GOAL(S) _____

_____

_____

**DAILY GOALS
ACHIEVED**

FLEXIBILITY · RELAXATION · MEDITATION

Activity Performed	Minutes
FLEXIBILITY · RELAXATION · MEDITATION TOTALS:	
COMMENTS:	

NUTRITIONAL INTAKE

Food Item	amt.	cal.	fat gms	protein gms	carbs gms	fiber gms
BREAKFAST:						
LUNCH:						
DINNER:						
SNACKS:						
INTAKE TOTALS:						

VITAMINS & SUPPLEMENTS

Type: _____

Qty: _____

Type: _____

Qty: _____

Type: _____

Qty: _____

Type: _____

Qty: _____

WATER INTAKE:

OF 8oz GLASSES

❑ ❑

❑ ❑

❑ ❑

❑ ❑

❑ ❑

COMMENTS · NOTES · PROGRESS

_____

_____

_____

_____

_____

DATE:_____ WEEK#:_____ DAY#:_____   WEIGHT:_____

ENERGY LEVELS: low ❑ med ❑ high ❑

Daily Workout Journal

Your
everyday
life offers
healthy ways
to exercise.
Taking
the stairs
instead of
the elevator,
riding a
bicycle to
work, or
parking
further from
your office
can help you
lose weight
and build
fitness.

CARDIOVASCULAR EXERCISE   STRETCHING/WARMUP: yes ❑ no ❑

Time	Exercise Type	Minutes	Distance	Pace/ Setting	Cal. Burned
CARDIO EXERCISE TOTALS:					

COMMENTS:

STRENGTH TRAINING   TARGET AREA: upper body ❑ lower body ❑ abs ❑

Exercise Type	Muscle Group	SET 1 Reps/Wt.	SET 2 Reps/Wt.	SET 3 Reps/Wt.	SET 4 Reps/Wt.
STRENGTH TRAINING TOTALS:					

COMMENTS:

OTHER · GROUP EXERCISE   STRETCHING/WARMUP: yes ❑ no ❑

Time	Exercise Type	Minutes	Cal. Burned
OTHER · GROUP EXERCISE TOTALS:			

COMMENTS:

DAILY GOAL(S)_____

_____

_____

**DAILY GOALS
ACHIEVED**

FLEXIBILITY · RELAXATION · MEDITATION

Activity Performed	Minutes
FLEXIBILITY · RELAXATION · MEDITATION TOTALS:	
COMMENTS:	

NUTRITIONAL INTAKE

Food Item	amt.	cal.	fat gms	protein gms	carbs gms	fiber gms
BREAKFAST:						
LUNCH:						
DINNER:						
SNACKS:						
INTAKE TOTALS:						

**VITAMINS &
SUPPLEMENTS**

Type:_____

Qty:_____

Type:_____

Qty:_____

Type:_____

Qty:_____

Type:_____

Qty:_____

WATER INTAKE:

OF 8OZ GLASSES

❑ ❑

❑ ❑

❑ ❑

❑ ❑

❑ ❑

COMMENTS · NOTES · PROGRESS

_____

_____

_____

_____

_____

_____

DATE:_____ WEEK#:_____ DAY#:_____ WEIGHT:_____

Helpful Tips

Daily Workout Journal

Although running a mile takes less time to accomplish than walking, both burn the same amount of calories.

CARDIOVASCULAR EXERCISE   STRETCHING/WARMUP: yes ☐ no ☐

Time	Exercise Type	Minutes	Distance	Pace/Setting	Cal. Burned
CARDIO EXERCISE TOTALS:					

COMMENTS:

STRENGTH TRAINING   TARGET AREA: upper body ☐ lower body ☐ abs ☐

Exercise Type	Muscle Group	SET 1 Reps/Wt.	SET 2 Reps/Wt.	SET 3 Reps/Wt.	SET 4 Reps/Wt.
STRENGTH TRAINING TOTALS:					

WORKOUT REMINDER:

_____

_____

_____

_____

COMMENTS:

OTHER·GROUP EXERCISE   STRETCHING/WARMUP: yes ☐ no ☐

Time	Exercise Type	Minutes	Cal. Burned
OTHER·GROUP EXERCISE TOTALS:			

COMMENTS:

DAILY GOAL(S)_____

_____

_____

DAILY GOALS
ACHIEVED

FLEXIBILITY · RELAXATION · MEDITATION

Activity Performed	Minutes
FLEXIBILITY · RELAXATION · MEDITATION TOTALS:	

COMMENTS:

NUTRITIONAL INTAKE

Food Item	amt.	cal.	fat gms	protein gms	carbs gms	fiber gms
BREAKFAST:						
LUNCH:						
DINNER:						
SNACKS:						
INTAKE TOTALS:						

VITAMINS & SUPPLEMENTS

Type:_____

Qty:_____

Type:_____

Qty:_____

Type:_____

Qty:_____

Type:_____

Qty:_____

WATER INTAKE:

OF 8OZ GLASSES

☐ ☐

☐ ☐

☐ ☐

☐ ☐

☐ ☐

COMMENTS · NOTES · PROGRESS

_____

_____

_____

_____

_____

_____

DATE:_____ WEEK#:_____ DAY#:_____   WEIGHT:_____

ENERGY LEVELS: low ☐ med ☐ high ☐

Daily Workout Journal

CARDIOVASCULAR EXERCISE   STRETCHING/WARMUP: yes ☐ no ☐

Time	Exercise Type	Minutes	Distance	Pace/ Setting	Cal. Burned
CARDIO EXERCISE TOTALS:					

COMMENTS:

STRENGTH TRAINING   TARGET AREA: upper body ☐ lower body ☐ abs ☐

Exercise Type	Muscle Group	SET 1 Reps/Wt.	SET 2 Reps/Wt.	SET 3 Reps/Wt.	SET 4 Reps/Wt.
STRENGTH TRAINING TOTALS:					

WORKOUT REMINDER:

_____

_____

_____

_____

_____

_____

COMMENTS:

_____

_____

_____

_____

_____

_____

OTHER · GROUP EXERCISE   STRETCHING/WARMUP: yes ☐ no ☐

Time	Exercise Type	Minutes	Cal. Burned
OTHER · GROUP EXERCISE TOTALS:			

COMMENTS:

DAILY GOAL(S) _____

_____

DAILY GOALS
ACHIEVED

FLEXIBILITY · RELAXATION · MEDITATION

Activity Performed	Minutes
FLEXIBILITY · RELAXATION · MEDITATION TOTALS:	
COMMENTS:	

NUTRITIONAL INTAKE

Food Item	amt.	cal.	fat gms	protein gms	carbs gms	fiber gms
BREAKFAST:						
LUNCH:						
DINNER:						
SNACKS:						
INTAKE TOTALS:						

VITAMINS & SUPPLEMENTS

Type: _____

Qty: _____

Type: _____

Qty: _____

Type: _____

Qty: _____

Type: _____

Qty: _____

WATER INTAKE:

OF 8oz GLASSES

❏ ❏

❏ ❏

❏ ❏

❏ ❏

❏ ❏

COMMENTS · NOTES · PROGRESS

_____

_____

_____

_____

_____

ENERGY LEVELS: low ☐ med ☐ high ☐

Helpful Tips

Daily Workout Journal

Visualizing yourself achieving your goals can help get you through difficult workout sessions and even help you reach new levels of fitness.

CARDIOVASCULAR EXERCISE   STRETCHING/WARMUP: yes ☐ no ☐

Time	Exercise Type	Minutes	Distance	Pace/Setting	Cal. Burned
CARDIO EXERCISE TOTALS:					

COMMENTS:

STRENGTH TRAINING   TARGET AREA: upper body ☐ lower body ☐ abs ☐

Exercise Type	Muscle Group	SET 1 Reps/Wt.	SET 2 Reps/Wt.	SET 3 Reps/Wt.	SET 4 Reps/Wt.
STRENGTH TRAINING TOTALS:					

WORKOUT REMINDER:

_____

_____

_____

_____

_____

_____

COMMENTS:

OTHER · GROUP EXERCISE   STRETCHING/WARMUP: yes ☐ no ☐

Time	Exercise Type	Minutes	Cal. Burned
OTHER · GROUP EXERCISE TOTALS:			

COMMENTS:

DAILY GOAL(S)_____

_____

_____

DAILY GOALS ACHIEVED

FLEXIBILITY · RELAXATION · MEDITATION

Activity Performed	Minutes
FLEXIBILITY · RELAXATION · MEDITATION TOTALS:	
COMMENTS:	

NUTRITIONAL INTAKE

Food Item	amt.	cal.	fat gms	protein gms	carbs gms	fiber gms
BREAKFAST:						
LUNCH:						
DINNER:						
SNACKS:						
INTAKE TOTALS:						

VITAMINS & SUPPLEMENTS

Type:_____

Qty:_____

Type:_____

Qty:_____

Type:_____

Qty:_____

Type:_____

Qty:_____

WATER INTAKE:

OF 8OZ GLASSES

❑ ❑

❑ ❑

❑ ❑

❑ ❑

❑ ❑

COMMENTS · NOTES · PROGRESS

_____

_____

_____

_____

_____

DATE:_____ WEEK#:_____ DAY#:_____   WEIGHT:_____

ENERGY LEVELS: low ☐ med ☐ high ☐

Helpful Tips

Daily Workout Journal

Exercise can boost your mental acuity by increasing the level of serotonin and other neurotransmitters in your brain.

CARDIOVASCULAR EXERCISE   STRETCHING/WARMUP: yes ☐ no ☐

Time	Exercise Type	Minutes	Distance	Pace/Setting	Cal. Burned
CARDIO EXERCISE TOTALS:					

COMMENTS:

STRENGTH TRAINING   TARGET AREA: upper body ☐ lower body ☐ abs ☐

Exercise Type	Muscle Group	SET 1 Reps/Wt.	SET 2 Reps/Wt.	SET 3 Reps/Wt.	SET 4 Reps/Wt.
STRENGTH TRAINING TOTALS:					

WORKOUT REMINDER:

_____

_____

_____

_____

_____

COMMENTS:

OTHER · GROUP EXERCISE   STRETCHING/WARMUP: yes ☐ no ☐

_____

_____

_____

Time	Exercise Type	Minutes	Cal. Burned
OTHER · GROUP EXERCISE TOTALS:			

COMMENTS:

FLEXIBILITY · RELAXATION · MEDITATION

Activity Performed	Minutes
FLEXIBILITY · RELAXATION · MEDITATION TOTALS:	

COMMENTS:

NUTRITIONAL INTAKE

Food Item	amt.	cal.	fat gms	protein gms	carbs gms	fiber gms
BREAKFAST:						
LUNCH:						
DINNER:						
SNACKS:						
INTAKE TOTALS:						

VITAMINS &
SUPPLEMENTS

Type: _____
Qty: _____

Type: _____
Qty: _____

Type: _____
Qty: _____

Type: _____
Qty: _____

WATER INTAKE:
OF 8oz GLASSES

❑ ❑
❑ ❑
❑ ❑
❑ ❑
❑ ❑

COMMENTS · NOTES · PROGRESS

_____
_____
_____
_____
_____

DATE:_____ WEEK#:_____ DAY#:_____ WEIGHT:_____

ENERGY LEVELS: low ☐ med ☐ high ☐

Daily Workout Journal

CARDIOVASCULAR EXERCISE   STRETCHING/WARMUP: yes ☐ no ☐

Exercise can
decrease
stress by
serving as a
distraction
from
everyday
problems.
Decreased
levels of
stress, in
turn, can lead
to improved
relationships
at work and
at home.

Time	Exercise Type	Minutes	Distance	Pace/Setting	Cal. Burned
CARDIO EXERCISE TOTALS:					

COMMENTS:

STRENGTH TRAINING   TARGET AREA: upper body ☐ lower body ☐ abs ☐

Exercise Type	Muscle Group	SET 1 Reps/Wt.	SET 2 Reps/Wt.	SET 3 Reps/Wt.	SET 4 Reps/Wt.
STRENGTH TRAINING TOTALS:					

COMMENTS:

OTHER · GROUP EXERCISE   STRETCHING/WARMUP: yes ☐ no ☐

Time	Exercise Type	Minutes	Cal. Burned
OTHER · GROUP EXERCISE TOTALS:			

COMMENTS:

FLEXIBILITY · RELAXATION · MEDITATION

Activity Performed	Minutes
FLEXIBILITY · RELAXATION · MEDITATION TOTALS:	

COMMENTS:

NUTRITIONAL INTAKE

Food Item	amt.	cal.	fat gms	protein gms	carbs gms	fiber gms
BREAKFAST:						
LUNCH:						
DINNER:						
SNACKS:						
INTAKE TOTALS:						

VITAMINS & SUPPLEMENTS

Type:
Qty:

Type:
Qty:

Type:
Qty:

Type:
Qty:

WATER INTAKE:

OF 8OZ GLASSES

❏ ❏
❏ ❏
❏ ❏
❏ ❏
❏ ❏

COMMENTS · NOTES · PROGRESS

DATE:_____ WEEK#:_____ DAY#:_____ WEIGHT:_____

ENERGY LEVELS: low ☐ med ☐ high ☐

Daily Workout Journal

Exercise
energizes
you. When
you exercise
your body
releases
endorphins,
naturally
produced
substances
that reduce
fatigue and
give you a
sense of well-
being.

CARDIOVASCULAR EXERCISE   STRETCHING/WARMUP: yes ☐ no ☐

Time	Exercise Type	Minutes	Distance	Pace/ Setting	Cal. Burned
CARDIO EXERCISE TOTALS:					

COMMENTS:

STRENGTH TRAINING   TARGET AREA: upper body ☐ lower body ☐ abs ☐

Exercise Type	Muscle Group	SET 1 Reps/Wt.	SET 2 Reps/Wt.	SET 3 Reps/Wt.	SET 4 Reps/Wt.
STRENGTH TRAINING TOTALS:					

COMMENTS:

OTHER · GROUP EXERCISE   STRETCHING/WARMUP: yes ☐ no ☐

Time	Exercise Type	Minutes	Cal. Burned
OTHER · GROUP EXERCISE TOTALS:			

COMMENTS:

DAILY GOAL(S) _____

DAILY GOALS
ACHIEVED

FLEXIBILITY · RELAXATION · MEDITATION

Activity Performed	Minutes
FLEXIBILITY · RELAXATION · MEDITATION TOTALS:	

COMMENTS:

NUTRITIONAL INTAKE

Food Item	amt.	cal.	fat gms	protein gms	carbs gms	fiber gms
BREAKFAST:						
LUNCH:						
DINNER:						
SNACKS:						
INTAKE TOTALS:						

VITAMINS &
SUPPLEMENTS

Type: _____
Qty: _____

Type: _____
Qty: _____

Type: _____
Qty: _____

Type: _____
Qty: _____

WATER INTAKE:
OF 8OZ GLASSES

❏ ❏

❏ ❏

❏ ❏

❏ ❏

❏ ❏

COMMENTS · NOTES · PROGRESS

DATE:_____ WEEK#:_____ DAY#:_____   WEIGHT:_____

ENERGY LEVELS: low ❏ med ❏ high ❏

Daily Workout Journal

Your fitness
routine need
not interfere
with your
relationships.
A weekly
hike or
bicycle ride,
for example,
can be a
great time to
bond with
your spouse,
children, or
friends.

CARDIOVASCULAR EXERCISE   STRETCHING/WARMUP: yes ❏ no ❏

Time	Exercise Type	Minutes	Distance	Pace/ Setting	Cal. Burned
CARDIO EXERCISE TOTALS:					

COMMENTS:

STRENGTH TRAINING   TARGET AREA: upper body ❏ lower body ❏ abs ❏

Exercise Type	Muscle Group	SET 1 Reps/Wt.	SET 2 Reps/Wt.	SET 3 Reps/Wt.	SET 4 Reps/Wt.
STRENGTH TRAINING TOTALS:					

COMMENTS:

OTHER · GROUP EXERCISE   STRETCHING/WARMUP: yes ❏ no ❏

Time	Exercise Type	Minutes	Cal. Burned
OTHER · GROUP EXERCISE TOTALS:			

COMMENTS:

**DAILY GOALS
ACHIEVED**

FLEXIBILITY · RELAXATION · MEDITATION

Activity Performed	Minutes
FLEXIBILITY · RELAXATION · MEDITATION TOTALS:	

COMMENTS:

NUTRITIONAL INTAKE

Food Item	amt.	cal.	fat gms	protein gms	carbs gms	fiber gms
BREAKFAST:						
LUNCH:						
DINNER:						
SNACKS:						
INTAKE TOTALS:						

VITAMINS & SUPPLEMENTS

Type:
Qty:

Type:
Qty:

Type:
Qty:

Type:
Qty:

WATER INTAKE:
OF 8OZ GLASSES

❑ ❑
❑ ❑
❑ ❑
❑ ❑
❑ ❑

COMMENTS · NOTES · PROGRESS

ENERGY LEVELS: low ☐ med ☐ high ☐

Helpful Tips

Daily Workout Journal

Track your progress toward fitness by placing a star or some other mark on your calendar for each day you work out.

CARDIOVASCULAR EXERCISE   STRETCHING/WARMUP: yes ☐ no ☐

Time	Exercise Type	Minutes	Distance	Pace/ Setting	Cal. Burned
CARDIO EXERCISE TOTALS:					

COMMENTS:

STRENGTH TRAINING   TARGET AREA: upper body ☐ lower body ☐ abs ☐

Exercise Type	Muscle Group	SET 1 Reps/Wt.	SET 2 Reps/Wt.	SET 3 Reps/Wt.	SET 4 Reps/Wt.
STRENGTH TRAINING TOTALS:					

WORKOUT REMINDER:

_____

_____

_____

_____

_____

_____

_____

_____

_____

COMMENTS:

OTHER · GROUP EXERCISE   STRETCHING/WARMUP: yes ☐ no ☐

Time	Exercise Type	Minutes	Cal. Burned
OTHER · GROUP EXERCISE TOTALS:			

COMMENTS:

DAILY GOAL(S)_____

_____

_____

FLEXIBILITY · RELAXATION · MEDITATION

Activity Performed	Minutes
FLEXIBILITY · RELAXATION · MEDITATION TOTALS:	
COMMENTS:	

NUTRITIONAL INTAKE

Food Item	amt.	cal.	fat gms	protein gms	carbs gms	fiber gms
BREAKFAST:						
LUNCH:						
DINNER:						
SNACKS:						
INTAKE TOTALS:						

VITAMINS & SUPPLEMENTS

Type:_____
Qty:_____

Type:_____
Qty:_____

Type:_____
Qty:_____

Type:_____
Qty:_____

WATER INTAKE:
OF 8OZ GLASSES

❏ ❏
❏ ❏
❏ ❏
❏ ❏
❏ ❏

COMMENTS · NOTES · PROGRESS

_____

_____

_____

_____

_____

_____

ENERGY LEVELS: low ☐ med ☐ high ☐

Daily Workout Journal

Helpful Tips

Keeping goals in mind can help you achieve them. Some people, for example, find it helpful to write their goals on a piece of paper and then put the paper where they will see it everyday.

CARDIOVASCULAR EXERCISE   STRETCHING/WARMUP: yes ☐ no ☐

Time	Exercise Type	Minutes	Distance	Pace/ Setting	Cal. Burned
CARDIO EXERCISE TOTALS:					

COMMENTS:

STRENGTH TRAINING   TARGET AREA: upper body ☐ lower body ☐ abs ☐

Exercise Type	Muscle Group	SET 1 Reps/Wt.	SET 2 Reps/Wt.	SET 3 Reps/Wt.	SET 4 Reps/Wt.
STRENGTH TRAINING TOTALS:					

COMMENTS:

WORKOUT REMINDER:

OTHER · GROUP EXERCISE   STRETCHING/WARMUP: yes ☐ no ☐

Time	Exercise Type	Minutes	Cal. Burned
OTHER · GROUP EXERCISE TOTALS:			

COMMENTS:

DAILY GOAL(S) _____

_____

_____

**DAILY GOALS
ACHIEVED**

FLEXIBILITY · RELAXATION · MEDITATION

Activity Performed	Minutes
FLEXIBILITY · RELAXATION · MEDITATION TOTALS:	
COMMENTS:	

NUTRITIONAL INTAKE

Food Item	amt.	cal.	fat gms	protein gms	carbs gms	fiber gms
BREAKFAST:						
LUNCH:						
DINNER:						
SNACKS:						
INTAKE TOTALS:						

VITAMINS & SUPPLEMENTS

Type: _____
Qty: _____

Type: _____
Qty: _____

Type: _____
Qty: _____

Type: _____
Qty: _____

WATER INTAKE:

OF 8oz GLASSES

❑ ❑
❑ ❑
❑ ❑
❑ ❑
❑ ❑

COMMENTS · NOTES · PROGRESS

_____

_____

_____

_____

_____

DATE:_____ WEEK#:_____ DAY#:_____   WEIGHT:_____

ENERGY LEVELS: low ☐   med ☐   high ☐

Helpful Tips

Daily Workout Journal

Joining a fitness group or participating in a team sport is an excellent way to exercise and maintain motivation.

CARDIOVASCULAR EXERCISE   STRETCHING/WARMUP: yes ☐   no ☐

Time	Exercise Type	Minutes	Distance	Pace/ Setting	Cal. Burned
CARDIO EXERCISE TOTALS:					

COMMENTS:

STRENGTH TRAINING   TARGET AREA: upper body ☐   lower body ☐   abs ☐

Exercise Type	Muscle Group	SET 1 Reps/Wt.	SET 2 Reps/Wt.	SET 3 Reps/Wt.	SET 4 Reps/Wt.
STRENGTH TRAINING TOTALS:					

WORKOUT REMINDER:

_____

_____

_____

_____

_____

_____

_____

_____

_____

_____

COMMENTS:

OTHER · GROUP EXERCISE   STRETCHING/WARMUP: yes ☐   no ☐

Time	Exercise Type	Minutes	Cal. Burned
OTHER · GROUP EXERCISE TOTALS:			

COMMENTS:

DAILY GOAL(S) _____

_____

_____

DAILY GOALS
ACHIEVED

FLEXIBILITY · RELAXATION · MEDITATION

Activity Performed	Minutes
FLEXIBILITY · RELAXATION · MEDITATION TOTALS:	
COMMENTS:	

NUTRITIONAL INTAKE

Food Item	amt.	cal.	fat gms	protein gms	carbs gms	fiber gms
BREAKFAST:						
LUNCH:						
DINNER:						
SNACKS:						
INTAKE TOTALS:						

VITAMINS & SUPPLEMENTS

Type: _____
Qty: _____

Type: _____
Qty: _____

Type: _____
Qty: _____

Type: _____
Qty: _____

WATER INTAKE:

OF 8OZ GLASSES

☐ ☐
☐ ☐
☐ ☐
☐ ☐
☐ ☐

COMMENTS · NOTES · PROGRESS

_____

_____

_____

_____

_____

ENERGY LEVELS: low ❏ med ❏ high ❏

Helpful Tips

Daily Workout Journal

You are more likely to work out regularly if your exercise partner is someone you see everyday, such as a co-worker or neighbor.

CARDIOVASCULAR EXERCISE STRETCHING/WARMUP: yes ❏ no ❏

Time	Exercise Type	Minutes	Distance	Pace/Setting	Cal. Burned
CARDIO EXERCISE TOTALS:					

COMMENTS:

STRENGTH TRAINING TARGET AREA: upper body ❏ lower body ❏ abs ❏

Exercise Type	Muscle Group	SET 1 Reps/Wt.	SET 2 Reps/Wt.	SET 3 Reps/Wt.	SET 4 Reps/Wt.
STRENGTH TRAINING TOTALS:					

WORKOUT REMINDER:

_____

_____

_____

_____

_____

COMMENTS:

OTHER · GROUP EXERCISE STRETCHING/WARMUP: yes ❏ no ❏

Time	Exercise Type	Minutes	Cal. Burned
OTHER · GROUP EXERCISE TOTALS:			

COMMENTS:

DAILY GOAL(S) _____

_____

_____

**DAILY GOALS
ACHIEVED**

FLEXIBILITY · RELAXATION · MEDITATION

Activity Performed	Minutes
FLEXIBILITY · RELAXATION · MEDITATION TOTALS:	
COMMENTS:	

NUTRITIONAL INTAKE

Food Item	amt.	cal.	fat gms	protein gms	carbs gms	fiber gms
BREAKFAST:						
LUNCH:						
DINNER:						
SNACKS:						
INTAKE TOTALS:						

**VITAMINS &
SUPPLEMENTS**

Type: _____
Qty: _____

Type: _____
Qty: _____

Type: _____
Qty: _____

Type: _____
Qty: _____

WATER INTAKE:

OF 8OZ GLASSES

❏ ❏
❏ ❏
❏ ❏
❏ ❏
❏ ❏

COMMENTS · NOTES · PROGRESS

_____

_____

_____

_____

_____

NUTRITIONAL FACTS ON POPULAR FOOD ITEMS

This section is a great resource for nutritional information on foods you may want to select for your weight loss program. It provides calories per serving, as well as the content in grams for protein, fats, carbohydrates, and fiber.

To use this section, look up a food item and its corresponding information. Then, log this data in your journal so that you can track your daily totals.

Common Items You Like to Eat

FOOD ITEM	Serving Size	Cal.	Fat	Protein	Carbs	Fiber

NUTRITIONAL INFORMATION

Nutrition values for fat, protein, carbohydrates, and fiber are listed in grams per serving.
Serving sizes and values are approximate.

FOOD ITEM	Serving Size	Cal.	Fat	Protein	Carbs	Fiber
A						
Alcohol, 100 proof	1 fl oz	82	0	0	0	0
Alcohol, 86 proof	1 fl oz	70	0	0	0	0
Alcohol, 90 proof	1 fl oz	73	0	0	0	0
Alcohol, 94 proof	1 fl oz	76	0	0	0	0
Alcohol, Beer, regular	12 fl oz	117	0.2	9.1	5.7	0
Alcohol, Daiquiri	8 fl oz	448	0	0	16.8	0
Alcohol, dessert wine, dry	1 glass	157	0	0.2	12	0
Alcohol, dessert wine, sweet	1 glass	165	0	0.2	14.1	0
Alcohol, liquors	1 fl oz	107	0.1	0	11.2	0
Alcohol, Pilsner Urquell	12 fl oz	156	0	1.8	16	0
Alcohol, pina colada	8 fl oz	440	4.8	1	57	0.4
Alcohol, Tequila Sunrise	8 fl oz	272	0	.8	28	0
Alfalfa seeds	1 tbsp	1	0	0.1	0.1	0.1
Almond butter, w/ salt	1 tbsp	101	9.5	2.4	3.4	0.6
Almond butter, w/o salt	1 tbsp	101	9.5	2.4	3.4	0.6
Almonds, roasted	1 oz (12 nuts)	169	15	6.2	5.5	3.3
Anchovies	3 oz	111	4.1	17.3	0	0
Apple juice	8 fl oz	120	0.2	0.2	28.8	0
Apples, w/o skin	1 medium	61	0.2	0.3	16	1.7
Apples, w/ skin	1 medium	72	0.2	0.4	19	3.3
Applesauce	1 cup	194	0.5	0.5	50.8	3.1
Apricots	1 apricot	17	0.1	0.5	3.9	0.7
Artichokes	1 artichoke	76	0.2	5.3	17	8.7
Arugula	1 cup	4	0.1	0.5	0.7	0.4
Asparagus	1 spear	2	0	0.3	0.5	0.3
Avocados	1 cup, cubes	240	22	3	12.8	10
B						
Bacon bits, meatless	1 tbsp	33	1.8	2.2	2	0.7
Bacon, Canadian, cooked	1 slice	43	2	5.8	0.3	0
Bacon, meatless	1 slice	16	1.5	0.5	0.3	0.1
Bacon, pork, cooked	1 slice	42	3.2	3	0.1	0
Bagels, cinnamon-raisin	1 bagel, 4" dia	244	1.5	8.7	49	2
Bagels, egg	1 bagel, 4" dia	292	2.2	11	55.6	2.4
Bagels, oat-bran	1 bagel, 4" dia	227	1	9.5	47	3.2
Bagels, plain	1 bagel, 4" dia	245	1.4	9.3	47	2
Bagels, deli gourmet style	1 bagel	370	3	13	71	2
Balsam pear	1 balsam pear	21	0.2	1.2	4.6	3.5
Bamboo shoots	1 cup	41	0.5	3.9	7.9	3.3
Banana chips	1 oz	147	9.5	0.7	16.6	2.2
Bananas	1 medium, 7"-8"	105	0.4	13	27	3
Barley	1 cup	651	4.2	23	135.2	31.8
Barley flour	1 cup	511	2.4	15.5	110.3	14.9
Barley, pearled, cooked	1 cup	193	0.7	3.6	44.3	6
Basil	5 leaves	1	0	0.1	0.1	0.1
Basil, dried	1 tsp	2	0	0.1	0.4	0.3
Bay leaf	1 tsp, crumbled	2	0.1	0	0.4	0.2
Beans, adzuki, cooked	1 cup	294	0.2	17	57	16.8
Beans, baked, canned, plain	1 cup	239	0.9	12.1	53.7	10.4
Beans, baked, canned, w/o salt	1 cup	266	1	12.1	52.1	13.9

FOOD ITEM	Serving Size	Cal.	Fat	Protein	Carbs	Fiber
B (cont.)						
Beans, baked, canned, w/ beef	1 cup	322	9.2	17	45	10
Beans, black, cooked	1 cup	227	0.9	15	40	15
Beans, cranberry, cooked	1 cup	241	0.8	16	43	18
Beans, fava, canned	1 cup	182	0.5	14	31	9.5
Beans, french, cooked	1 cup	228	1.3	12	43	17
Beans, great northern, cooked	1 cup	209	0.8	15	37	12
Beans, kidney, cooked	1 cup	225	0.9	15	40	11
Beans, lima, cooked	1 cup	216	0.7	15	39	13
Beans, lima, canned	1 can	190	0.4	12	36	11
Beans, mung, cooked	1 cup	212	0.7	14	39	15
Beans, mungo, cooked	1 cup	189	1	13.5	33	11.5
Beans, navy, cooked	1 cup	255	1	15	47	19
Beans, pink, cooked	1 cup	252	0.8	15	47	18
Beans, pinto, cooked	1 cup	245	1	15	44	15
Beans, small white, cooked	1 cup	254	1	16	46	18
Beans, snap, green, cooked	1 cup	44	0.3	2	10	4
Beans, snap, yellow, cooked	1 cup	44	0.3	2	10	4
Beans, white, cooked	1 cup	249	0.6	17	45	11
Beans, yellow	1 cup	255	2	16	48	18
Beechnuts, dried	1 oz	163	14.2	1.8	9.5	0
Beef, choice short rib, cooked	3 oz	400	35.6	18.3	0	0
Beef bologna	1 slice	88	8	3.3	0.6	0
Beef jerky, chopped	1 piece	81	5.1	6.6	2.2	0.4
Beef sausage, precooked	1 link	134	11.6	6	1	0
Beef stew, canned	1 serving	218	12.5	11.5	15.7	3.5
Beef, tri-tip roast, roasted	3 oz	174	9.4	22.2	0	0
Beef, brisket, lean and fat, roasted	3 oz	328	26.8	20	0	0
Beef, brisket, lean, roasted	3 oz	206	10.8	25.3	0	0
Beef, chuck, arm roast, lean & fat, braised	3 oz	283	19.6	23.3	0	0
Beef, chuck, arm roast, lean, braised	3 oz	179	6.5	28.1	0	0
Beef, chuck, top blade, raw	3 oz	138	7.5	16.5	0	0
Beef, cured breakfast strips	3 slices	276	26.4	8.5	0.5	0
Beef, cured, corned, canned	3 oz	213	12.8	23	0	0
Beef, cured, dried	1 serving	43	0.5	8.7	0.8	0
Beef, cured, luncheon meat	1 slice	31	0.9	5.4	0	0
Beef, flank, raw	1 oz	47	2.4	6	0	0
Beef, ground patties, frozen	3 oz	240	19.7	14.5	0	0
Beef, ground, 70% lean, raw	1 oz	94	8.5	4.1	0	0
Beef, ground, 80% lean, raw	1 oz	72	5.7	4.9	0	0
Beef, ground, 95% lean, raw	1 oz	39	1.4	6.1	0	0
Beef, rib, large end, boneless, raw	1 oz	94	8.3	4.5	0	0
Beef, rib, shortribs, boneless, raw	1 oz	110	10.3	4.1	0	0
Beef, rib, whole, boneless, raw	1 oz	91	7.9	4.6	0	0
Beef, rib-eye, small end, raw	1 oz	78	6.3	5	0	0
Beef, round, bottom, raw	1 oz	56	3.4	5.9	0	0
Beef, round, eye, raw	1 oz	49	2.5	6.1	0	0
Beef, round, full cut, raw	1 oz	55	3.4	5.8	0	0
Beef, round, tip, raw	1 oz	56	3.6	5.5	0	0
Beef, round, top, raw	1 oz	48	2.3	6.2	0	0
Beef, shank crosscuts, raw	1 oz	50	2.8	5.8	0	0

NUTRITIONAL INFORMATION

Nutrition values for fat, protein, carbohydrates, and fiber are listed in grams per serving.
Serving sizes and values are approximate.

FOOD ITEM	Serving Size	Cal.	Fat	Protein	Carbs	Fiber
B (cont.)						
Beef, short loin, porterhouse, raw	1 oz	73	5.7	5.1	0	0
Beef, short loin, t-bone, raw	1 oz	66	4.8	5.4	0	0
Beef, short loin, top, raw	1 oz	66	4.5	5.8	0	0
Beef, sirloin, tri-tip, raw	1 oz	50	3	5.8	0	0
Beef, tenderloin, raw	1 oz	70	5.1	5.6	0	0
Beef, top sirloin, raw	1 oz	61	4	5.6	0	0
Beer, light	12 fl oz	110	12	4.8	7	0
Beer, nonalcoholic	12 fl oz	80	1	0	70	0
Beer, regular	12 fl oz	140	12	0.9	10	0.7
Beets	1 beet	35	0	2	8	4
Bratwurst, chicken	1 serving	148	8.7	16.3	0	0
Bratwurst, pork	1 serving	281	24.8	11.7	2.1	0
Bratwurst, veal	1 serving	286	26.6	11.8	0	0
Bread stuffing, dry mix, prepared	1/2 cup	178	8.6	3	22	3
Bread, banana	1 slice	196	6.3	2.5	32.7	0.7
Bread, corn	1 piece	188	6	4.3	28.8	1.4
Bread, cracked-wheat	1 slice	65	1	2.2	11.8	1
Bread, french	1 slice	70	1	3	15	1
Bread, garlic	1 slice	160	10	3	14	1
Bread, Irish soda	1 oz	82	1.4	1.9	15.9	0.7
Bread, pita	2 oz	150	1	3	30	0
Bread, pumpernickel	1 slice	75	1	3	15	2
Bread, raisin	1 slice	80	1.5	2	15	1
Bread, rice bran	1 oz	69	1.3	2.5	12.3	1.4
Bread, sandwich slice	1 slice	70	1	2	13	1
Bread, sourdough	1 slice	100	1	2	20	1
Broad beans, cooked	1 cup	187	0.6	13	33.4	9.2
Brownies	1 brownie	220	13	1	27	1
Buckwheat	1 cup	583	5.8	22.5	121.6	17
Buckwheat flour	1 cup	402	3.7	15.1	84.7	12
Buckwheat groats, roasted, cooked	1 cup	155	1	5.6	33.5	4.5
Buffalo, raw	1 oz	28	0.4	5.8	0	0
Burbot, raw	3 oz	77	0.7	16.4	0	0
Burdock root	1 cup	85	0.2	1.8	20.5	3.9
Butter, whipped, w/ salt	1 tbsp	67	7.6	0.1	0	0
Butternuts, dried	1 oz	174	16	7	3	1.3
C						
Cabbage, common	1 cup, shredded	17	1	1	4	1.6
Cabbage, pak choi	1 cup, shredded	9	0.1	1.1	1.5	0.7
Cabbage, pe-tsai	1 cup, shredded	12	0.2	0.9	2.5	0.9
Cake, angel food	1 slice	180	4	2	36	2
Cake, boston cream pie	1 slice	260	9	1	32	0
Cake, carrot	1 slice	310	16	1	39	0
Cake, cheesecake	1 slice	500	30	4	50	0
Cake, chocolate	1 slice	270	13	1	36	1
Cake, chocolate mousse	1 slice	250	10	1	35	1
Cake, devil's food	1 slice	270	13	2	35	0
Cake, pineapple upside-down	1 piece	367	13.9	4	58.1	0.9
Cake, pound	1 slice	320	16	2	38	0

FOOD ITEM	Serving Size	Cal.	Fat	Protein	Carbs	Fiber
C (cont.)						
Cake, sponge cake w/ cream, berries	1 slice	325	8	25	38	1
Cake, yellow	1 slice	260	11	2	36	1
Candy, butterscotch	5 pieces	120	2.5	0	20	0
Candy, caramels	1 piece	30	1	3	6	1
Candy, carob	1 bar	470	27.3	7.1	49	3.3
Candy, chocolate fudge	1 oz.	125	5	0	18	0
Candy, chocolate mints	1 mint	45	1	0	9	0
Candy, milk chocolate w/ almonds	1.5 oz.	216	14	3.7	21	2.5
Candy, chocolate-coated peanut butter bites	1 piece	45	2.5	1	4	0
Candy, chocolate-coated peanuts	12 peanuts	160	11	20	15	7
Candy, gumdrops	4 pieces	130	0	0	31	0
Candy, hard candy	1 piece	18	0	0	5	0
Candy, jelly beans	12 beans	100	0	0	24	0
Candy, licorice	1 piece	30	0	0	7	0
Candy, lollipop	1 lollipop	20	0	0	5	0
Candy, milk chocolate bar	1.5 oz.	235	13	3.3	26	1.5
Candy, mints	1 mint	30	0	0	7	0
Cantaloupe	1 cup, cubed	54	0.3	1.3	13.1	1.4
Cardoon	1 cup, shredded	36	0.2	1.2	8.7	2.8
Carrots	1 medium	65	0	1	15	4
Cashew butter, w/ salt	1 tbsp.	94	7.9	2.8	4.4	0.3
Cashew nuts	1 oz.	157	12.4	5.2	8.6	0.9
Cassava	1 cup	330	0.6	2.8	78.4	3.7
Celeraic	1 cup	66	0.5	2.3	14.4	2.8
Chard, swiss	1 cup	7	0.1	0.6	1.3	0.6
Cheese, american	1 slice	110	9	5	1	0
Cheese, brick	1 oz.	100	8	31	0	0
Cheese, brie	1 oz.	95	8	50	1	0
Cheese, camembert	1 oz.	90	7	49	1	0
Cheese, cheddar	1 oz.	110	9	33	0.5	0
Cheese, colby jack	1 oz.	110	9	31	0.5	0
Cheese, cottage, 2%	1 cup	203	4	31	8	0
Cheese, edam	1 oz.	100	8	7	0	0
Cheese, feta	1 oz.	100	8	21	1	0
Cheese, goat	1 oz.	128	10.1	8.7	0.6	0
Cheese, goat, semisoft	1 oz.	103	8.5	6.1	0.7	0
Cheese, goat, soft	1 oz.	76	6	5.3	0.3	0
Cheese, gouda	1 oz.	100	8	7	0.5	0
Cheese, monterey jack	1 oz.	110	9	32	0	0
Cheese, mozzarella	1 oz.	90	7	25	0.5	0
Cheese, parmesan, hard	1 oz.	110	7	10	1	0
Cheese, parmesan, shredded	1 tbsp.	22	1.5	2	0	0
Cheese, provolone	1 oz.	100	8	34	1	0
Cheese, queso	2 tbsp.	110	9	28	2	0
Cheese, ricotta	2 tbsp.	50	3.5	28	1	0
Cheese, roquefort	1 oz.	105	9	6	0.5	0
Cheese, swiss	1 oz.	110	9	36	1	0
Cherries, sour	8 pieces	30	0	1	7	2
Cherries, sweet	8 pieces	30	0	2	7	2
Chewing gum	1 piece	25	0	0	5	0

NUTRITIONAL INFORMATION

Nutrition values for fat, protein, carbohydrates, and fiber are listed in grams per serving.
Serving sizes and values are approximate.

FOOD ITEM	Serving Size	Cal.	Fat	Protein	Carbs	Fiber
C (cont.)						
Chicken, breast, w/ skin	1/2 breast	249	13.4	30.2	0	0
Chicken, breast, w/o skin	1/2 breast	130	1.5	27.2	0	0
Chicken, capons, boneless	1/2 capon	1459	74	184	0	0
Chicken, capons, giblets, cooked	1 cup	238	8	38	1	0
Chicken, cornish game hen, roasted	1/2 bird	336	24	29	0	0
Chicken, cornish game hen, meat only	1 bird	295	9	51	0	0
Chicken, dark meat, w/o skin	1 cup diced	287	14	38	0	0
Chicken, drumstick, w/ skin	1 drumstick	118	6.3	14.1	0	0
Chicken, drumstick, w/o skin	1 drumstick	74	2.1	12.8	0	0
Chicken, leg, w/ skin	1 leg	312	20.2	30.3	0	0
Chicken, leg, w/o skin	1 leg	156	5	26.2	0	0
Chicken, light meat, w/o skin	1 cup diced	214	6	38	0	0
Chicken, thigh, w/ skin	1 thigh	198	14.3	16.2	0	0
Chicken, thigh, w/o skin	1 thigh	82	2.7	13.6	0	0
Chicken, wing, w/ skin	1 wing	109	7.8	9	0	0
Chicken, wing, w/o skin	1 wing	37	1	6.4	0	0
Chickpeas, cooked	1 cup	269	4	15	45	12.5
Chicory greens	1 cup, chopped	41	0.5	3.1	8.5	7.2
Chicory roots	1/2 cup	33	0.1	0.6	7.9	0
Chicory, witloof	1/2 cup	8	0	0.4	1.8	1.4
Chili con carne w/ beans	1 cup	298	13	17.5	28	10
Chili powder	1 tsp	8	0.4	0.3	1.4	0.9
Chili w/ beans, canned	1 cup	287	14	14.5	30.5	11
Chili w/o beans, canned	1 cup	194	6.5	17	18	3
Chinese chestnuts	1 oz	64	0.3	1.2	13.9	0
Chives	1 tbsp, chopped	1	0	0.1	0.1	0.1
Chocolate chip crisped rice bar	1 bar	115	3.8	1.4	20.7	0.6
Chocolate chips	1/4 cup	210	12	3	24	1
Chocolate milkshake, ready-to-drink	8 fl oz	181	5	8	26	1
Chocolate, semi sweet bars, baking	1 oz	160	8	3	20	1
Chocolate, unsweetened baking squares	1 square	144	15	3.7	8.6	4.8
Chorizo, pork and beef	1 link	273	23	14.5	1.1	0
Chow mein noodles	1 cup	237	13.8	3.8	25.9	1.8
Cinnamon, ground	1 tsp	6	0.1	0.1	1.8	1.2
Cisco	3 oz	83	1.6	16.1	0	0
Citrus fruit drink, from concentrate	8 fl oz	124	0.1	0.5	30	0.8
Clam, mixed species, raw	1 large	15	0.2	2.6	0.5	0
Cloves, ground	1 tsp	7	0.4	0.1	1.3	0.7
Cocktail mix, nonalcoholic	1 fl oz	103	0	0.1	25.8	0
Cocoa mix, powder	1 serving	113	1.1	1.7	24	1
Cocoa mix, powder, unsweetened	1 tbsp	12	0.7	1.1	2.9	1.8
Coconut meat	1 cup, shredded	283	26.8	2.7	12.2	7.2
Coconut milk	1 cup	552	57.2	5.5	13.3	5.3
Coffee, brewed, decaf	1 cup	0	0	0.2	0	0
Coffee, brewed, regular	1 cup	2	0	0.3	0	0
Coffee, café au lait	8 fl oz	65	2.5	1	6	0
Coffee, cappuccino	8 fl oz	70	4	1	6	0
Coffee, espresso	1 shot	4	0	0	1	0
Coffee, instant, decaf	1 tsp	0	0	0	0	0
Coffee, instant, regular	1 tsp, dry	2	0	0.1	0.4	0

NUTRITIONAL INFORMATION

Nutrition values for fat, protein, carbohydrates, and fiber are listed in grams per serving.
Serving sizes and values are approximate.

C (cont.)

FOOD ITEM	Serving Size	Cal.	Fat	Protein	Carbs	Fiber
Coffee, latte	8 fl oz.	100	5	0	8	0
Coffee, mocha	8 fl oz.	180	12	1	16	0
Coffeecake	2.5 oz.	230	7	3.8	38	3.8
Coleslaw	1/2 cup	41	1.6	0.8	7.4	0.9
Collards	1 cup, chopped	11	0.2	0.9	2	1.3
Conch, baked or broiled	1 cup, sliced	165	1.5	33.4	2.2	0
Cookies, animal crackers	1 cookie	22	0.7	0.3	3.6	0.1
Cookies, brownies	3.5 oz.	430	25	1	52	1.2
Cookies, butter	1 cookie	23	0.9	0.3	3.4	0
Cookies, chocolate chip, deli fresh baked	1 cookie	275	15	0	37.5	1
Cookies, chocolate chip, commercial	1 cookie	130	6.9	0.9	16.7	0.9
Cookies, chocolate chip, refrigerated dough	1 portion	128	5.9	1.3	17.8	0.4
Cookies, chocolate wafers	1 wafer	26	0.8	0.4	4.3	0.2
Cookies, fig bars	1 cookie	150	3.1	1.6	30.5	2
Cookies, fudge	1 cookie	73	0.8	1.1	16.4	0.6
Cookies, gingersnap	1 cookie	29	0.7	0.4	5.4	0.2
Cookies, graham, plain or honey	2 1/2" square	30	0.7	0.5	5.3	0.2
Cookies, marshmallow w/ chocolate coating	1 cookie	118	4.7	1.1	19	0.6
Cookies, molasses	1 cookie	138	4.1	1.8	23.6	0.3
Cookies, oatmeal	1 cookie	238	8.8	2.5	37.5	2
Cookies, oatmeal w/ raisins	1 cookie	238	8.8	2.5	37.5	2
Cookies, oatmeal, commercial, iced	1 cookie	123	4.8	1.4	18.4	0.6
Cookies, oatmeal, refrigerated dough	1 portion	68	3	0.9	9.5	0.4
Cookies, peanut butter sandwich	1 cookie	67	3	1.2	9.2	0.3
Cookies, peanut butter, refrigerated dough	1 portion	73	4	1.3	8.3	0.2
Cookies, sugar	1 cookie	66	3.3	0.8	8.4	0.2
Cookies, sugar wafers w/ cream filling	1 wafer	46	2.2	0.4	6.3	0.1
Cookies, sugar, refrigerated dough	1 portion	113	5.4	1.1	15.3	0.2
Cookies, vanilla wafers	1 wafer	28	1.2	0.3	4.3	0.1
Coriander leaves	9 sprigs	5	0.1	0.4	0.7	0.6
Corn flour, yellow	1 cup	416	4.3	10.6	86.9	0
Corn, sweet, white	1 ear	77	1.1	2.9	17.1	2.4
Corn, sweet, yellow	1 ear	77	1.1	2.9	17.1	2.4
Corn, sweet, white, cream style	1 cup	184	1	4.5	46.4	3.1
Corn, sweet, yellow, cream style	1 cup	184	1	4.5	46.4	3.1
Cornnuts	1 oz.	126	4.4	2.4	20.4	2
Cornstarch	1 cup	488	0.1	0.3	116.8	1.2
Couscous, cooked	1 cup	176	0.2	6	36.5	0.1
Cowpeas (black-eyed peas), cooked	1 cup	160	0.6	5.2	33.5	8.2
Cowpeas, catjang, cooked	1 cup	200	1.2	14	34.7	6.2
Cowpeas, leafy tips	1 cup, chopped	10	0.1	1.5	1.7	0
Crab, alaska king, raw	1 leg	144	1	31.5	0	0
Crab, blue, canned	1 cup	134	1.6	27.7	0	0
Crab, dungeness, cooked	1 crab	140	1.6	28.4	1.2	0
Crabapples	1 cup, sliced	84	0.3	0.4	21.9	0
Crackers w/ cheese filling	6 crackers	191	9.5	3.5	22.9	0.7
Crackers w/ peanut butter filling	6 cracker	193	9.8	4.8	22.1	1.3
Crackers, cheese, regular	6 crackers	312	15.7	6.3	36.1	1.5
Crackers, graham	1 cracker	30	0.5	6	5	2
Crackers, matzo, plain	1 matzo	112	0.4	2.8	23.7	0.9

NUTRITIONAL INFORMATION

Nutrition values for fat, protein, carbohydrates, and fiber are listed in grams per serving.
Serving sizes and values are approximate.

FOOD ITEM	Serving Size	Cal.	Fat	Protein	Carbs	Fiber
C (cont.)						
Crackers, matzo, whole-wheat	1 matzo	100	0.4	3.7	22.4	3.3
Crackers, melba toast	1 cup	129	1.1	4	25.3	2.1
Crackers, milk	1 cracker	50	1.7	0.8	7.7	0.2
Crackers, regular	1 cup, bite size	311	15.7	4.6	37.8	1
Crackers, rusk toast	1 rusk	41	0.7	1.4	7.2	0
Crackers, rye	1 cracker	37	0.1	1.1	8.8	2.5
Crackers, saltines	1 cracker	20	0.1	0.5	4.1	0.1
Crackers, soda	1 cracker	60	2	6	10	2
Crackers, wheat	1 cracker	9	0.4	0.1	1.3	0.1
Crackers, wheat, sandwich w/ peanut butter	1 cracker	35	1.8	0.9	3.7	0.3
Crackers, whole-wheat	1 cracker	18	0.7	0.3	2.7	0.4
Cranberries	1 cup, whole	44	0.1	0.4	11.6	4.4
Cranberry juice cocktail	1 cup	144	0.3	0	36.4	0.3
Cranberry-apple juice	1 cup	174	0.1	0.2	44.3	0.2
Cranberry-grape juice	1 cup	137	0.2	0.5	34.3	0.2
Crayfish, wild, raw	8 crayfish	21	0.3	4.3	0	0
Cream cheese	1 tbsp	51	5.1	1.1	0.4	0
Cream of tartar	1 tsp	8	0	0	1.8	0
Cream, half & half	1 tbsp	20	1.7	0.4	0.6	0
Cream, heavy whipping	1 cup, fluid	821	88.1	4.9	6.6	0
Crepes	1 crepe	120	6	2	14	1
Croissants, apple	1 croissant	145	5	4.2	21.1	1.4
Croissants, butter	1 croissant	115	6	2.3	13	0.7
Croissants, cheese	1 croissant	174	8.8	3.9	19.7	1.1
Croutons, plain	1 cup	122	2	3.6	22.1	1.5
Croutons, seasoned	1 cup	186	7.3	4.3	25.4	2
Cucumber	1 cucumber	45	0.3	2	10.9	1.5
Cucumber, peeled	1 cup, sliced	14	0.2	0.7	2.6	0.8
Cumin seed	1 tsp	8	0.5	0.4	0.9	0.2
Currants, black	1 cup	71	0.5	1.6	17.2	0
Currants, red & white	1 cup	63	0.2	1.6	15.5	4.8
Curry powder	1 tsp	7	0.3	0.3	1.2	0.7
D						
Dandelion greens	1 cup, chopped	25	0.4	1.5	5.1	1.9
Danish pastry, cheese, 4 1/4" diameter	1 pastry	266	15.5	5.7	26.4	0.7
Danish pastry, cinnamon, 4 1/4" diameter	1 pastry	262	14.5	4.5	29	0.8
Danish pastry, fruit, 4 1/4" diameter	1 pastry	263	13	3.8	33.9	1.3
Danish pastry, nut, 4 1/4" diameter	1 pastry	280	16.4	4.6	29.7	1.3
Danish pastry, raspberry, 4 1/4" diameter	1 pastry	263	13.1	3.8	33.9	1.3
Deer, ground, raw	1 oz	45	2	6.2	0	0
Deer, raw	1 oz	34	0.7	6.5	0	0
Doughnuts, chocolate coated or frosted	1 doughnut	133	8.7	1.4	13.4	0.6
Doughnuts, chocolate, sugared or glazed	1 doughnut	250	11.9	2.7	34.4	1.3
Doughnuts, french crullers	1 cruller	169	7.5	1.3	24.4	0.5
Doughnuts, plain	1 doughnut, stick	219	11.9	2.6	25.8	0.8
Doughnuts, wheat, sugared or glazed	1 doughnut	101	5.4	1.8	11.9	0.6
Duck liver, raw	1 liver	60	2	8.2	1.6	0
Duck, meat only, roasted	1/2 duck	444	24.7	51.9	0	0
Duck, white pekin, breast w/skin, roasted	1/2 breast	242	13	29.4	0	0

NUTRITIONAL INFORMATION

Nutrition values for fat, protein, carbohydrates, and fiber are listed in grams per serving.
Serving sizes and values are approximate.

FOOD ITEM	Serving Size	Cal.	Fat	Protein	Carbs	Fiber
D (cont.)						
Duck, skinless, raw	1/2 duck	400	18	55.4	0	0
Durian	1 cup, chopped	357	13	3.6	65.8	9.2
E						
Eclairs w/ chocolate glaze	1 éclair	293	17.6	7.2	27.1	0.7
Eel, mixed species, raw	3 oz	156	9.9	15.7	0	0
Egg noodles, cooked	1 cup	213	2.3	7.6	39.7	1.8
Egg substitute, liquid	1 tbsp	13	0.5	1.9	0.1	0
Egg white, fried	1 large	92	7	6.3	0.4	0
Egg white, raw	1 large	17	0.1	3.6	0.2	0
Egg yolk, raw	1 large	53	4.4	2.6	0.6	0
Egg, hard-boiled	1 cup, chopped	211	14.4	17.1	1.5	0
Egg, omelette	1 large	93	7.3	6.5	0.4	0
Egg, poached	1 large	74	4.9	6.3	0.4	0
Egg, raw	1 large	85	5.8	7.3	0.4	0
Egg, scrambled	1 cup	365	26.9	24.4	4.8	0
Eggnog	8 fl oz	343	19	9.6	34	0
Eggplant	1 eggplant	110	0.9	4.6	26.1	15.6
Elderberries	1 cup	106	0.7	1	26.7	10.2
Elk, ground, raw	1 oz	49	2.5	6.2	0	0
Elk, raw	1 oz	31	0.4	6.5	0	0
Endive	1 head	87	1	6.4	17.2	15.9
English muffins, plain	1 muffin	134	1	4.4	26.2	1.5
English muffins, cinnamon-raisin	1 muffin	139	1.5	4.2	48.7	1.7
English muffins, wheat	1 muffin	127	1.1	5	25.5	2.6
English muffins, whole-wheat	1 muffin	134	1.4	5.8	26.6	4.4
English muffins, whole-wheat/multigrain	1 muffin	155	1.2	6	30.5	1.8
European chestnuts, peeled	1 oz	56	0.4	0.5	12.5	0
European chestnuts, unpeeled	1 oz	60	0.6	0.7	12.9	2.3
F						
Farina, cooked	1 cup	471	0.1	3.3	24.4	0.7
Fast food, biscuit w/ egg	1 biscuit	373	22.1	11.6	31.9	0.8
Fast food, biscuit w/ egg & bacon	1 biscuit	458	31.1	17	28.6	0.8
Fast food, biscuit w/ egg, bacon & cheese	1 biscuit	477	31.4	16.3	33.4	0.1
Fast food, biscuit w/ sausage	1 biscuit	485	31.8	12.1	40	1.4
Fast food, caramel sundae	1 sundae	304	9.3	7.3	49.3	0
Fast food, cheeseburger, large, double patty	1 sandwich	704	43.7	38	39.7	1
Fast food, cheeseburger, large, single patty	1 sandwich	563	32.9	28.2	38.4	1
Fast food, corndog	1 corndog	460	18.9	16.8	55.8	1
Fast food, croissant w/ egg, cheese	1 croissant	368	24.7	12.8	24.3	1
Fast food, croissant w/ egg, cheese, bacon	1 croissant	413	28.4	16.2	23.6	1
Fast food, croissant w/ egg, cheese, sausage	1 croissant	523	38.2	20.3	24.7	1
Fast food, Danish pastry, cheese	1 pastry	353	24.6	5.8	28.7	1.5
Fast food, Danish pastry, cinnamon	1 pastry	349	16.7	4.8	46.9	1.5
Fast food, Danish pastry, fruit	1 pastry	335	15.9	4.8	45.1	1.5
Fast food, fish sandwich w/ tartar sauce	1 sandwich	431	22.8	16.9	41	1
Fast food, french toast sticks	5 pieces	513	29	8.3	57.9	2.7
Fast food, fried chicken, boneless	6 pieces	285	18.1	15	15.7	0.9
Fast food, hamburger, large, double patty	1 sandwich	540	26.6	34.3	40.3	2.1

NUTRITIONAL INFORMATION

Nutrition values for fat, protein, carbohydrates, and fiber are listed in grams per serving.
Serving sizes and values are approximate.

FOOD ITEM	Serving Size	Cal.	Fat	Protein	Carbs	Fiber
F (cont.)						
Fast food, hamburger, large, single patty	1 sandwich	425	20.9	23	36.7	2.1
Fast food, hot fudge sundae	1 sundae	284	8.6	5.6	47.7	0
Fast food, hot dog w/ chili	1 hot dog	296	13.4	13.5	31.3	1
Fast food, hot dog, plain	1 hot dog	242	14.5	10.4	18	1
Fast food, McDonald's Big Mac® w/ cheese	1 serving	560	30	25	46	3.1
Fast food, McDonald's Big Mac® w/o cheese	1 serving	495	25.4	23.2	43.3	2.7
Fast food, McDonald's cheeseburger	1 serving	310	12	15	35	1
Fast food, McDonald's Chicken McGrill®	1 serving	400	16	27	38	3
Fast food, McDonald's Crispy Chicken	1 serving	500	23	24	50	3
Fast food, McDonald's Filet-o-Fish®	1 serving	400	18	14	42	1
Fast food, McDonald's french fries	1 medium	350	11	4	47	5
Fast food, McDonald's hamburger	1 serving	260	9	13	33	1
Fast food, McDonald's 1/4 Pounder®,cheese	1 serving	510	25	29	43	3
Fast food, McDonald's 1/4 Pounder®	1 serving	420	18	24	40	3
Fast food, onion rings, 8-9 rings	1 portion	276	15.5	3.7	31.3	3.3
Fast food, strawberry sundae	1 sundae	268	7.8	6.3	44.6	0
Fast food, submarine sandwich w/ cold cuts	1 submarine 6"	456	18.6	21.8	51	4
Fast food, submarine sandwich w/ roast beef	1 submarine 6"	410	13	28.6	44.3	4
Fast food, submarine sandwich w/ tuna	1 submarine 6"	584	28	29.7	55.4	4
Fast food, vanilla soft-serve w/ cone	1 cone	164	6.1	3.9	24.1	0.1
Fennel bulb	1 cup, sliced	27	0.2	1.1	6.3	2.7
Fennel seed	1 tbsp	20	0.9	0.9	3	2.3
Fenugreek seed	1 tbsp	36	0.7	2.6	6.5	2.7
Figs	1 medium	37	0.2	0.4	9.6	1.5
Figs, dried	1 fig	21	0.01	0.3	5.3	0.8
Fireweed leaves	1 cup, chopped	24	0.6	1.1	4.4	2.4
Fish oil, cod liver	1 tbsp	123	13.6	0	0	0
Fish oil, herring	1 tbsp	123	13.6	0	0	0
Fish oil, menhaden	1 tbsp	123	13.6	0	0	0
Fish oil, salmon	1 tbsp	123	13.6	0	0	0
Fish oil, sardine	1 tbsp	123	13.6	0	0	0
Fish, bluefin tuna, raw	3 oz	122	4.2	19.8	0	0
Fish, bluefish, raw	3 oz	105	3.6	17	0	0
Fish, butterfish, raw	3 oz	124	6.8	14.7	0	0
Fish, carp, raw	3 oz	108	4.8	15.2	0	0
Fish, catfish, raw	3 oz	81	2.4	13.9	0	0
Fish, cod, atlantic, raw	3 oz	70	0.6	15.1	0	0
Fish, croaker, atlantic, raw	3 oz	88	2.7	15.1	0	0
Fish, flatfish, raw	3 oz	77	1	16	0	0
Fish, gefilte fish	1 piece	35	0.7	3.8	3.1	0
Fish, grouper, mixed species, raw	3 oz	78	0.9	16.5	0	0
Fish, haddock, raw	3 oz	74	0.6	16.1	0	0
Fish, halibut, raw	3 oz	94	1.9	17.7	0	0
Fish, herring, atlantic, raw	3 oz	134	7.7	15.3	0	0
Fish, herring, pacific, raw	3 oz	166	11.8	13.9	0	0
Fish, mackerel, atlantic, raw	3 oz	174	11.8	15.8	0	0
Fish, mackerel, king, raw	3 oz	89	1.7	17.2	0	0
Fish, mackerel, pacific, raw	3 oz	134	6.7	17.1	0	0
Fish, mackerel, spanish, raw	3 oz	118	5.4	16.4	0	0
Fish, milkfish, raw	3 oz	126	5.7	17.5	0	0

Nutrition values for fat, protein, carbohydrates, and fiber are listed in grams per serving.
Serving sizes and values are approximate.

FOOD ITEM	Serving Size	Cal.	Fat	Protein	Carbs	Fiber
F (cont.)						
Fish, monkfish, raw	3 oz.	65	1.3	12.3	0	0
Fish, ocean perch, atlantic, raw	3 oz.	80	1.4	15.8	0	0
Fish, perch, mixed species, raw	3 oz.	77	0.8	16.5	0	0
Fish, pike, northern, raw	3 oz.	75	0.6	16.4	0	0
Fish, pollock, atlantic, raw	3 oz.	78	0.8	16.5	0	0
Fish, pout, ocean, raw	3 oz.	67	0.8	14.1	0	0
Fish, rainbow smelt, raw	3 oz.	82	2.1	15	0	0
Fish, rockfish, pacific, raw	3 oz.	80	1.3	15.9	0	0
Fish, roe, mixed species, raw	1 tbsp.	20	0.9	3.1	0.2	0
Fish, sablefish, raw	3 oz.	166	13	11.4	0	0
Fish, salmon, atlantic, farmed, raw	3 oz.	156	9.2	16.9	0	0
Fish, salmon, atlantic, wild, raw	3 oz.	121	5.4	16.9	0	0
Fish, salmon, chinook, raw	3 oz.	152	8.9	16.9	0	0
Fish, salmon, pink, raw	3 oz.	99	2.9	16.9	0	0
Fish, sea bass, mixed species, raw	3 oz.	82	1.7	15.7	0	0
Fish, seatrout, mixed species, raw	3 oz.	88	3.1	14.2	0	0
Fish, shad, raw	3 oz.	167	11.7	14.4	0	0
Fish, skipjack tuna, raw	3 oz.	88	0.9	18.7	0	0
Fish, snapper, mixed species, raw	3 oz.	85	1.1	17.4	0	0
Fish, striped bass, raw	3 oz.	82	2	15.1	0	0
Fish, striped mullet	3 oz.	99	3.2	16.4	0	0
Fish, sturgeon, mixed species, raw	3 oz.	89	3.4	13.7	0	0
Fish, swordfish, raw	3 oz.	103	3.4	16.8	0	0
Fish, trout, mixed species, raw	3 oz.	126	5.6	17.7	0	0
Fish, white sucker, raw	3 oz.	78	2	14.2	0	0
Fish, whitefish, raw	3 oz.	114	5	16.2	0	0
Fish, wolffish, atlantic, raw	3 oz.	82	2	14.9	0	0
Fish, yellowfin tuna, raw	3 oz.	93	0.9	19.8	0	0
Fish, yellowtail, mixed species, raw	3 oz.	124	4.5	19.7	0	0
Flan, caramel custard	5 1/2 oz.	303	12	4	43	0
Flaxseed	1 tbsp.	59	4.1	2.3	4.1	3.3
Flaxseed oil	1 tbsp.	120	13.6	0	0	0
Frankfurter	1 serving	151	13.4	5.3	2.2	0
Frankfurter, beef	1 frankfurter	188	16.9	6.4	2.3	0
Frankfurter, beef & pork	1 frankfurter	174	15.8	6.6	1	1.4
Frankfurter, chicken	1 frankfurter	116	8.8	5.8	3.1	0
Frankfurter, meat	1 frankfurter	151	13.4	5.3	2.2	0
Frankfurter, meatless	1 frankfurter	163	9.6	13.7	5.4	2.7
Frankfurter, pork	1 frankfurter	204	18	9.7	0.2	0.1
Frankfurter, turkey	1 frankfurter	102	8	6.4	0.7	0
French fries, frozen, unprepared, 18 fries	1 serving	170	6.7	2.8	27.7	3.4
French toast, frozen, ready-to-heat	1 piece	126	3.6	4.3	18.9	0.6
Frosting, creamy chocolate	2 tbsp.	164	7.3	0.5	26.1	0.4
Frosting, creamy vanilla	2 tbsp.	160	6.3	0	25.6	0
Frozen yogurt, chocolate, soft-serve	1/2 cup	115	4.3	2.9	17.9	1.6
Frozen yogurt, vanilla, soft-serve	1/2 cup	117	4	2.9	17.4	0
Fruit cocktail, canned	1 cup	229	0.2	1	59.5	2.9
Fruit punch, prepared from concentrate	8 fl oz.	124	0.5	0.2	30.2	0.2
Fruit salad, canned in syrup	1 cup	186	0.2	0.9	48.7	2.6
Fruit salad, canned in water	1 cup	74	0.2	0.9	19.3	2.5

NUTRITIONAL INFORMATION

Nutrition values for fat, protein, carbohydrates, and fiber are listed in grams per serving.
Serving sizes and values are approximate.

FOOD ITEM	Serving Size	Cal.	Fat	Protein	Carbs	Fiber
G						
Garden cress, raw	1 cup	16	0.3	1.3	2.7	0.6
Garlic	1 clove	4	0	0.2	1	0.1
Garlic powder	1 tsp.	9	0	0.5	2	0.3
Gelatin dessert mix, prepared w/ water	1/2 cup	84	0	1.6	19.1	0
Gin, 80 Proof	1 fl oz.	73	0	0	0	0
Ginger root	1 tsp.	2	0	0	0.4	0
Ginger, ground	1 tsp.	6	0.1	0.2	1.3	0.2
Ginkgo nuts	1 oz.	52	0.5	1.2	10.7	0
Ginkgo nuts, dried	1 oz.	99	0.6	2.9	20.5	0
Goose liver, raw	1 liver	125	4	15.4	5.9	0
Goose, meat & skin, roasted	1 cup chopped	427	30.7	35.2	0	0
Goose, meat only, roasted	1 cup chopped	340	18.1	41.4	0	0
Gourd, white-flowered	1 gourd	108	0.2	4.8	26.1	0
Granola bars, hard, plain	1 bar	134	5.6	2.9	18.3	1.5
Granola bars, soft, plain	1 bar	126	4.9	2.1	19.1	1.3
Grape juice	8 fl oz.	160	0	0	40	0
Grapefruit	1/2 fruit	50	0	1	12	3
Grapefruit juice, sweetened	8 fl oz.	125	0	0	32.6	0
Grapefruit juice, unsweetened	8 fl oz.	91	0.2	1.2	21.5	0
Grapes, canned, heavy syrup	1 cup	187	0.3	1.2	50.3	1.5
Grapes, red or green	1 cup	106	0.2	1.1	27.9	1.4
Gravy, mushroom, canned	1 can	149	8.1	3.8	16.3	1.2
Gravy, au jus, canned	1 can	48	0.6	3.6	7.5	0
Gravy, beef, canned	1 can	154	6.9	10.9	14	1.2
Gravy, chicken, canned	1 can	235	17	5.8	16.2	1.2
Gravy, turkey, canned	1 can	152	6.2	7.7	15.2	1.2
Guacamole dip	2 tbsp.	50	4	12	4	0
Guavas	1 fruit	37	0.5	1.4	7.8	3
H						
Ham, chopped	1 slice	50	2.9	4.6	1.2	0
Ham, minced	1 slice	55	4.3	3.4	0.4	0
Ham, sliced	1 slice	46	2.4	4.6	1.1	0.4
Hazlenuts, dry roasted	1 oz.	183	17.7	4.2	5	2.7
Hazlenuts, blanched	1 oz.	178	17.3	3.9	4.8	3.1
Hominy, canned, white	1 cup	119	1.5	2.4	23.5	4.1
Hominy, canned, yellow	1 cup	115	1.4	2.4	22.8	4
Honey	1 tbsp.	64	0	0.1	17.3	0
Honeydew melons	1 cup, diced	61	0.2	0.9	15.5	1.4
Horseradish	1 tsp.	2	0	0.1	0.6	0.2
Hot chocolate	8 fl oz.	200	10	9	25	3
Hummus	1 tbsp.	23	1.3	1.1	2	0.8
Hush puppies	1 hush puppy	74	2.9	1.7	10.1	0.6
I						
Ice cream cone, rolled or sugar type	1 cone	40	0.4	0.8	8.4	0.4
Ice cream cone, wafer or cake type	1 cone	17	0.3	0.3	3.2	0.1
Ice cream, chocolate	1/2 cup	143	7.3	2.5	18.6	0.6
Ice cream, strawberry	1/2 cup	127	5.5	2.1	18.2	0.6
Ice cream, vanilla	1/2 cup	144	7.9	2.5	16.9	0.5

NUTRITIONAL INFORMATION

Nutrition values for fat, protein, carbohydrates, and fiber are listed in grams per serving.
Serving sizes and values are approximate.

FOOD ITEM	Serving Size	Cal.	Fat	Protein	Carbs	Fiber
I (cont.)						
Iced tea, presweetened	8 fl oz.	100	0	0	25	0
Iced tea, unsweetened	8 fl oz.	2	0	0	0	0
Italian seasoning	1 tsp.	4	0	0	1	0
J						
Jams and preserves	1 tbsp.	56	0	0.1	13.8	0.2
Japanese chestnuts	1 oz.	44	0.2	0.6	9.9	0
Japanese soba noodles, cooked	1 cup	113	0.1	5.7	24.4	1.7
Japanese ramen noodles, packaged, dry	1 serving	195	7.3	4	28	1
Jellies	1 tbsp.	55	0	0	14.4	0.2
K						
Kale	1 cup, chopped	34	0.5	2.2	6.7	1.3
Kiwifruit	1 medium	45	0	2	11	5
Kumquats	1 fruit	13	0.2	0.4	3	1.2
L						
Lamb, cubed, raw	1 oz.	38	1.5	5.7	0	0
Lamb, foreshank, raw	1 oz.	57	3.8	5.4	0	0
Lamb, ground, raw	1 oz.	80	6.6	4.7	0	0
Lamb, leg, shank half, raw	1 oz.	52	3.3	5.4	0	0
Lamb, leg, sirloin half, raw	1 oz.	74	5.9	4.9	0	0
Lamb, leg, whole, choice, raw	1 oz.	65	4.8	5.1	0	0
Lamb, loin, choice, raw	1 oz.	79	6.4	4.9	0	0
Lamb, rib, choice, raw	1 oz.	97	8.7	4.3	0	0
Lamb, shoulder, arm, raw	1 oz.	69	5.4	4.9	0	0
Lamb, shoulder, blade, raw	1 oz.	69	5.4	4.8	0	0
Lamb, shoulder, whole, raw	1 oz.	69	5.4	4.8	0	0
Lard	1 tbsp.	115	12.8	0	0	0
Leeks	1 leek	54	0.3	1.3	12.6	1.6
Lemon juice	1 cup	61	0	0.9	21.1	1
Lemon juice, canned or bottled	1 tbsp.	3	0	0.1	1	0.1
Lemon pepper seasoning	1 tsp.	7	0	0	1	0
Lemonade powder	1 scoop	102	0	0	26.9	0
Lemonade, pink concentrate, prepared	8 fl oz.	99	0	0.2	25.9	0
Lemonade, white concentrate, prepared	8 fl oz.	131	0.1	0.2	34	0.2
Lemons w/ peel	1 fruit	22	0.3	1.3	11.6	5.1
Lentils, cooked	1 cup	230	0.7	17.8	39.8	15.6
Lentils, sprouted, raw	1 cup	82	0.4	6.9	17	0
Lettuce, green leaf	1 cup, shredded	5	0.1	0.5	1	0.5
Lettuce, iceberg	1 cup, shredded	10	0.1	0.7	2.2	0.9
Lettuce, red leaf	1 cup, shredded	3	0	0.2	0.4	0.2
Lettuce, romaine	1 cup, shredded	8	0.1	0.6	1.5	1
Lime juice	1 cup	62	0.2	1	20.7	1
Limes	1 fruit	20	0.1	0.5	7.1	1.9
Liverwurst, pork	1 slice	59	5.1	2.5	0.4	0
Lobster, northern, raw	1 lobster	135	1.3	28.2	0.8	0
Luncheon meat, beef, loaved	1 oz.	87	7.4	4.1	0.8	0
Luncheon meat, beef, thin sliced	1 oz.	50	1.1	8	1.6	0
Luncheon meat, meatless slices	1 slice	26	1.6	2.5	0.6	0

NUTRITIONAL INFORMATION

Nutrition values for fat, protein, carbohydrates, and fiber are listed in grams per serving.
Serving sizes and values are approximate.

FOOD ITEM	Serving Size	Cal.	Fat	Protein	Carbs	Fiber
L (cont.)						
Luncheon meat, pork & chicken, minced	1 oz.	56	3.9	4.3	0.4	0
Luncheon meat, pork & ham, minced	1 oz.	88	7.45	3.75	1.3	0
Luncheon meat, pork or beef	1 oz.	99	9	3.5	0.6	0
Luncheon meat, pork, canned	1 oz.	95	8.6	3.5	0.6	0
Luncheon meat, pork, ham & chicken, minced	1 oz.	87	7.6	3.7	0.8	0
Luncheon sausage, pork & beef	1 oz.	74	5.9	4.3	0.4	0
M						
Macadamia nuts	1 oz. (10-12 nuts)	203	21.5	2.2	3.6	2.3
Macaroni and cheese, commercial, prepared	1 cup	259	2.6	11.3	47.5	1.5
Macaroni, cooked	1 cup	197	0.9	6.6	39.6	1.8
Malt drink mix, dry	3 heaping tsp.	87	1.7	2.4	15.9	0.2
Malt beverage	8 fl oz.	144	0.2	0.7	32.2	0
Mangos	1 fruit	135	0.6	1.1	35.2	3.7
Maraschino cherries	1 cherry	8	0	0	2.1	0.2
Margarine, fat free spread	1 tbsp.	6	0.4	0	0.6	0
Margarine, stick	1 tbsp.	100	11.2	0	0.3	0
Margarine, stick, unsalted	1 tbsp.	102	11.4	0.1	0.1	0
Margarine, tub	1 tbsp.	102	11.4	0.1	0.1	0
Martini	1 fl oz.	69	0	0	0.6	0
Mayonnaise	1 tbsp.	100	11	0	0	0
Milk, 1% low fat	1 cup	102	2.4	8.2	12.2	0
Milk, 2% low fat	1 cup	138	4.9	9.7	13.5	0
Milk, buttermilk, cultured, reduced fat	1 cup	137	4.9	10	13	0
Milk, chocolate	1 cup	208	8.5	7.9	25.9	2
Milk, dry, nonfat, instant	1/3 cup dry	82	0.1	8	12	0
Milk, evaporated	1/2 cup	169	9.5	8.5	12.6	0
Milk, skim or nonfat	1 cup	83	0.2	8.3	12.2	0
Milk, canned, sweetened condensed	1 cup	982	26.6	24.2	166.5	0
Milk, whole	1 cup	146	7.9	7.9	11	0
Milkshake, dry mix, vanilla	1 envelope packet	69	0.5	4.9	11.1	0.3
Millet	1 cup	756	8.4	22	145.7	17
Miso soup	1 cup	547	16.5	32.1	72.8	14.
Mixed nuts	1 cup	814	70.5	23.7	34.7	12.
Molasses	1 tablespoon	58	0	0	15	0
Muffins, apple bran	1 muffin	300	3	1	61	1
Muffins, banana nut	1 muffin	480	24	3	60	2
Muffins, blueberry	1 muffin	313	7.3	6.2	54.2	2.9
Muffins, chocolate chip	1 muffin	510	24	2	69	4
Muffins, corn	1 muffin	345	9.5	6.6	57.5	3.8
Muffins, oat bran	1 muffin	305	8.3	7.9	54.5	5.2
Muffins, plain	1 muffin	242	9.1	3.8	36.3	1.5
Mushrooms	1 cup, pieces	15	0.2	2.2	2.3	0.8
Mushrooms, enoki	1 large	2	0	0.1	0.4	0.1
Mushrooms, oyster	1 large	55	0.8	6.1	9.2	3.6
Mushrooms, portobello	1 large	0	0	0	0	0
Mushrooms, shiitake	1 mushroom	11	0	0.3	2.7	0.4
Mussels, blue, raw	1 cup	129	3.4	17.8	5.5	0
Mustard greens	1 cup, chopped	15	0.1	1.5	2.7	1.8
Mustard seed, yellow	1 tbsp.	53	3.2	2.8	3.9	1.6

NUTRITIONAL INFORMATION

Nutrition values for fat, protein, carbohydrates, and fiber are listed in grams per serving.
Serving sizes and values are approximate.

FOOD ITEM	Serving Size	Cal.	Fat	Protein	Carbs	Fiber
M (cont.)						
Mustard spinach	1 cup, chopped	33	0.5	3.3	5.9	4.2
Mustard, prepared, yellow	1 tsp.	3	0.2	0.2	0.4	0.2
N						
Natto (fermented soybeans)	1 cup	371	19.3	31	25.1	9.5
Nectarines	1 fruit	60	0.4	1.4	14.3	2.3
New Zealand spinach	1 cup, chopped	8	0.1	0.8	1.4	0
Nutmeg, ground	1 tsp.	12	0.8	0.1	1.1	0.5
O						
Oat bran	1 cup	231	6.6	16.3	62.2	14.5
Oatmeal, instant, prepared w/ water	1 cup	129	2.1	5.4	22.4	3.7
Oil, canola	1 tbsp.	124	14	0	0	0
Oil, canola & soybean	1 tbsp.	119	14	0	0	0
Oil, coconut	1 tbsp.	120	13.6	0	0	0
Oil, corn, peanut & olive	1 tbsp.	120	13.6	0	0	0
Oil, olive	1 tbsp.	119	13.5	0	0	0
Oil, peanut	1 tbsp.	119	13.5	0	0	0
Oil, sesame	1 tbsp.	120	13.6	0	0	0
Oil, soy	1 tbsp.	120	13.6	0	0	0
Oil, vegetable, almond	1 tbsp.	120	13.6	0	0	0
Oil, vegetable, cocoa butter	1 tbsp.	120	13.6	0	0	0
Oil, vegetable, coconut	1 tbsp.	117	13.6	0	0	0
Oil, vegetable, grapeseed	1 tbsp.	120	13.6	0	0	0
Oil, vegetable, hazelnut	1 tbsp.	120	13.6	0	0	0
Oil, vegetable, nutmeg butter	1 tbsp.	120	13.6	0	0	0
Oil, vegetable, palm	1 tbsp.	120	13.6	0	0	0
Oil, vegetable, poppyseed	1 tbsp.	120	13.6	0	0	0
Oil, vegetable, rice bran	1 tbsp.	120	13.6	0	0	0
Oil, vegetable, sheanut	1 tbsp.	120	13.6	0	0	0
Oil, vegetable, tomatoseed	1 tbsp.	120	13.6	0	0	0
Oil, vegetable, walnut	1 tbsp.	1927	218	0	0	0
Okra	1 cup	31	0.1	2	7	3.2
Onion powder	1 tsp.	8	0	0.2	1.9	0.1
Onions	1 cup, chopped	67	0.1	1.5	16.2	2.2
Onions, sweet	1 onion	106	0.3	2.7	25	3
Orange juice	8 fl oz	109	0.6	1.9	25	0.5
Orange marmalade	1 tbsp.	49	0	0.1	13.3	0.1
Oranges	1 large	86	0.2	1.7	21.6	4.4
Oregano, dried	1 tsp, ground	6	0.2	0.2	1.2	0.8
Oyster, eastern, raw	3 oz.	50	1.3	4.4	4.6	0
Oyster, pacific, raw	3 oz.	69	1.9	8	4.2	0
P						
Pancakes, blueberry	1 pancake	84	3.5	2.3	11	0
Pancakes, buttermilk	1 pancake	86	3.5	2.6	10.9	0
Pancakes, plain, dry mix	1 pancake	74	1	2	13.9	0.5
Papayas	1 cup, cubed	55	0.2	0.9	13.7	2.5
Paprika	1 tsp.	6	0.3	0.3	1.2	0.8
Parsley	1 cup	22	0.5	1.8	3.8	2

NUTRITIONAL INFORMATION

Nutrition values for fat, protein, carbohydrates, and fiber are listed in grams per serving.
Serving sizes and values are approximate.

FOOD ITEM	Serving Size	Cal.	Fat	Protein	Carbs	Fiber
P (cont.)						
Parsley, dried	1 tsp	1	0	0.1	0.2	0.1
Parsnips	1 cup, sliced	100	0.4	1.6	23.9	6.5
Passion fruit	1 fruit	17	0.1	0.4	4.2	1.9
Pasta, corn, cooked	1 cup	176	1	3.6	39	6.7
Pasta, plain, cooked	1 cup	197	0.9	6.6	39.6	2.4
Pasta, spinach, cooked	1 cup	195	1.4	7.6	37.5	2.4
Pastrami, turkey	1 oz	40	1.8	5.2	0.5	0
Pate de foie gras	1 tbsp	60	5.7	1.5	0.6	0
Pate, chicken liver, canned	1 tbsp	26	1.7	1.7	0.9	0
Pate, goose liver, canned	1 tbsp	60	5.7	1.5	0.6	0
Peaches	1 large	61	0.4	1.4	15	2.4
Peaches, canned	1 cup, halved	59	0.1	1.1	14.9	3.2
Peanut butter, chunky	2 tbsp	188	16	7.7	6.9	2.6
Peanut butter, smooth	2 tbsp	188	16.1	8	6.3	1.9
Peanuts, dry roasted w/ salt	1 oz	166	14	6.7	6.1	2.3
Peanuts, raw	1 oz	161	13.9	7.3	4.5	2.4
Pears	1 pear	121	0.3	0.8	32.3	6.5
Pears, asian	1 pear	116	0.6	1.4	29.3	9.9
Pears, canned	1 cup	71	0.1	0.5	19.1	3.9
Peas, green, fresh, cooked	1 cup	134	0.3	8.5	25	8.8
Peas, green, frozen, cooked	1 cup	125	0.4	8.2	22.8	8.8
Peas, split, cooked	1 cup	231	0.7	16.3	41.3	16.3
Pecans	1 oz. (20 halves)	196	20.4	2.6	3.9	2.7
Pepper, black	1 tsp	5	0.1	0.2	1.4	0.6
Pepper, red or cayenne	1 tsp	6	0.3	0.2	1	0.5
Pepperoni	15 slices	135	11.7	5.9	1.2	0
Peppers, chili, green	1 cup	29	0.4	1	6.4	2.4
Peppers, chili, red	1 pepper	18	0.2	0.8	4	0.7
Peppers, chili, sun-dried	1 pepper	2	0	0.1	0.4	0.2
Peppers, jalapeno	1 pepper	4	0.1	0.2	0.8	0.4
Peppers, sweet, green	1 medium	24	0.2	1	5.5	2
Peppers, sweet, red	1 medium	31	0.3	1.1	7.2	2.4
Peppers, sweet, yellow	1 medium	32	0.2	1.2	7.5	1.1
Persimmons	1 fruit	32	0.1	0.2	8.4	0
Pheasant, boneless, raw	1/2 pheasant	724	37.2	90.8	0	0
Pheasant, breast, skinless, boneless, raw	1/2 breast	242	5.9	44.4	0	0
Pheasant, leg, skinless, boneless, raw	1 leg	143	4.6	23.8	0	0
Pheasant, skinless, raw	1/2 pheasant	468	12.8	83	0	0
Pickle relish, sweet	1 tbsp	20	0.1	0.1	5.3	0.2
Pickle, sour	1 large 4"	15	0.3	0.4	3.1	1.6
Pickle, sweet	1 large 4"	158	0.3	0.5	42.9	1.5
Pickles, dill	1 large 4"	24	0.2	0.8	5.5	1.6
Pie crust, graham cracker, baked	1 pie crust	1037	52.3	8.8	136.9	3.2
Pie, apple	1 piece	411	19.4	3.7	57.5	0
Pie, blueberry	1 piece	290	12.5	2.2	43.6	1.3
Pie, cherry	1 piece	325	13.8	2.5	49.7	1
Pie, lemon meringue	1 piece	303	9.8	1.7	53.3	1.4
Pie, pecan	1 piece	452	20.9	4.5	64.6	4
Pie, pumpkin	1 piece	229	10.4	4.3	29.8	2.9
Pine nuts	1 oz. (167 kernels)	191	19.3	3.8	3.7	1

NUTRITIONAL INFORMATION

Nutrition values for fat, protein, carbohydrates, and fiber are listed in grams per serving.
Serving sizes and values are approximate.

P (cont.)

FOOD ITEM	Serving Size	Cal.	Fat	Protein	Carbs	Fiber
Pineapple	1 fruit	227	0.6	2.5	59.6	6.6
Pineapple, canned	1 slice	15	0	0.2	3.9	0.4
Pita bread, whole wheat	1 pita	170	1.7	6.4	35.2	4.8
Pistachio nuts	1 oz (49 kernels)	161	13	6	7.6	2.9
Pizza, cheese	1 slice (3.7 oz.)	250	10	11	29	2
Pizza, pepperoni	1 slice (3.7 oz.)	288	15.2	11.7	26.1	1.7
Plantains	1 medium	218	0.7	2.3	57.1	4.1
Plums	1 fruit	30	0.2	0.5	7.5	0.9
Plums, canned	1 plum	19	0	0.2	5.1	0.4
Polenta	1/2 cup	220	2	2	24	1
Pomegranates	1 fruit	105	0.5	1.5	26.4	0.9
Popcorn cakes	1 cake	38	0.3	1	8	0.3
Popcorn, air-popped	1 cup	31	0.3	1	6.2	1.2
Popcorn, caramel-coated	1 oz	122	3.6	1.1	22.4	1.5
Popcorn, cheese	1 cup	58	3.7	1	5.7	1.1
Popcorn, oil-popped	1 cup	55	3.1	1	6.3	1.1
Popovers, dry mix	1 oz	105	1.2	2.9	20	0.5
Poppy seed	1 tsp	15	1.3	0.5	0.7	0.3
Pork, cured, breakfast strips, cooked	3 slices	156	12.4	9.8	0.3	0
Pork, cured, ham, extra lean, canned	3 oz	116	4.1	17.9	0.4	0
Pork, cured, ham, patties	1 patty	205	18.4	8.3	1.1	0
Pork, cured, ham, extra lean, cooked	3 oz	140	6.5	18.6	0.4	0
Pork, cured, salt pork, raw	1 oz	212	22.8	1.4	0	0
Pork, fresh ground, cooked	3 oz	252	17.6	21.8	0	0
Pork, leg, rump half, cooked	3 oz	214	12.1	24.5	0	0
Pork, leg, shank half, cooked	3 oz	246	17	21.5	0	0
Pork, leg, whole, cooked	3 oz	232	14.9	22.8	0	0
Pork, loin, blade, cooked	3 oz	275	20.9	20.1	0	0
Pork, loin, center loin, cooked	3 oz	199	11.4	22.3	0	0
Pork, loin, center rib, cooked	3 oz	214	12.8	22.9	0	0
Pork, loin, sirloin, cooked	3 oz	176	8	24.2	0	0
Pork, loin, tenderloin, cooked	3 oz	147	5.1	23.6	0	0
Pork, loin, top loin, cooked	3 oz	192	9.7	24.4	0	0
Pork, loin, whole, cooked	3 oz	211	12.4	23	0	0
Pork, shoulder, arm, cooked	3 oz	238	18.1	17.3	0	0
Pork, shoulder, blade, cooked	3 oz	229	16	19.6	0	0
Pork, shoulder, whole, cooked	3 oz	248	18.2	19.8	0	0
Pork, spareribs, cooked	3 oz	337	25.7	24.7	0	0
Potato chips, barbecue	1 oz	139	9.2	2.2	14.9	1.2
Potato chips, cheese	1 oz	141	7.7	2.4	16.3	1.5
Potato chips, salted	1 oz	152	9.8	1.9	15	1.3
Potato chips, sour cream & onion	1 oz	151	9.6	2.3	14.6	1.5
Potato chips, reduced fat	1 oz	134	5.9	2	18.9	1.7
Potato chips, unsalted	1 oz	152	9.8	2	15	1.4
Potato flour	1 cup	571	0.5	11	132.9	9.4
Potato salad	1 cup	358	20.5	6.7	27.9	3.2
Potatoes	1 medium	164	0.2	4.3	37.2	4.7
Potatoes, baked, w/ skin	1 medium	160	0.2	4.3	36.5	3.8
Potatoes, baked, w/o skin	1 medium	143	0.2	2.8	33.3	3.3
Potatoes, mashed	1 cup	237	8.9	3.9	35.2	3.2

NUTRITIONAL INFORMATION

Nutrition values for fat, protein, carbohydrates, and fiber are listed in grams per serving.
Serving sizes and values are approximate.

FOOD ITEM	Serving Size	Cal.	Fat	Protein	Carbs	Fiber
P (cont.)						
Potatoes, red	1 medium	153	0.3	4	33.9	3.6
Potatoes, russet	1 medium	168	0.2	4.6	38.5	2.8
Potatoes, scalloped	1 cup	211	9	7	26.4	4.7
Potatoes, white	1 medium	149	0.2	3.6	33.5	5.1
Pretzels, hard, plain, salted	1 oz	108	0.9	2.6	22.4	0.9
Prune juice	8 fl oz	180	0	2	43	3
Pudding, banana	1/2 cup	154	2.5	4	29	0
Pudding, chocolate	1/2 cup	154	2.8	4.6	27.7	0
Pudding, coconut cream	1/2 cup	157	3.3	4.2	28.2	0.1
Pudding, lemon	1/2 cup	157	2.5	4	29.7	0
Pudding, rice	1/2 cup	163	2.4	4.8	30.6	0.1
Pudding, tapioca	1/2 cup	154	2.4	4.2	28.7	0
Pudding, vanilla	1/2 cup	148	2.5	4.3	27.2	0
Pumpkin	1 cup	30	0.1	1.2	7.5	0.6
Pumpkin pie mix	1 cup	281	0.4	2.9	71.3	22.
Pumpkin, canned	1 cup	83	0.7	2.7	19.8	7.1
R						
Rabbit, cooked	3 oz	167	6.8	24.7	0	0
Radicchio	1 cup, shredded	9	0.1	0.6	1.8	0.4
Radishes	1 cup, sliced	19	0.1	0.8	3.9	1.9
Raisins	1 1/2 oz	129	0.2	1.3	34	1.6
Raisins, golden	1 1/2 oz	130	0.2	1.4	34.1	1.7
Raspberries	1 cup	64	0.8	1.5	14.7	8
Rhubarb	1 cup, diced	26	0.2	1.1	5.5	2.2
Rice cakes, brown rice, corn	1 cake	35	0.3	0.8	7.3	0.3
Rice cakes, brown rice, multigrain	1 cake	35	0.3	0.8	7.2	0.3
Rice cakes, brown rice, plain	1 cake	35	0.3	0.7	7.3	0.4
Rice, brown, cooked	1 cup	218	1.6	4.5	45.8	3.5
Rice, white, cooked	1 cup	242	0.3	4.4	53.2	0.6
Rice, wild	1 cup	166	0.5	6.5	35	3
Rolls, dinner	1 roll	136	3.1	3.6	22.9	0.8
Rolls, dinner, wheat	1 roll	117	2.7	3.7	19.7	1.6
Rolls, dinner, whole-wheat	1 roll	114	2	3.7	21.9	3.2
Rolls, french	1 roll	119	1.8	3.7	21.5	0.1
Rolls, hamburger or hotdog	1 roll	120	1.9	4.1	21.3	0.9
Rolls, hard (incl. kaiser)	1 roll	126	1.8	4.2	22.6	1
Rolls, pumpernickel	1 roll	119	1.2	4.6	22.7	2.3
Rosemary	1 tsp	1	0	0	0.1	0.1
Rosemary, dried	1 tsp	4	0.2	0.1	0.8	0.5
Rum, 80 proof	1 fl oz	64	0	0	0	0
Rutabagas	1 cup, cubed	50	0.3	1.7	11.4	3.5
Rye	1 cup	566	4.2	24.9	117.9	24.
Rye flour, dark	1 cup	415	3.4	18	88	28.
Rye flour, light	1 cup	374	1.4	8.6	81.8	14.
Rye flour, medium	1 cup	361	1.8	9.6	79	14.
S						
Sage, ground	1 tsp	2	0.1	0.1	0.4	0.3
Sake	1 fl oz	39	0	0.1	1.5	0

NUTRITIONAL INFORMATION

Nutrition values for fat, protein, carbohydrates, and fiber are listed in grams per serving.
Serving sizes and values are approximate.

FOOD ITEM	Serving Size	Cal.	Fat	Protein	Carbs	Fiber
S (cont.)						
Salad dressing, 1000 island	1 tbsp.	58	5.5	0.2	2.3	0.1
Salad dressing, bacon & tomato	1 tbsp.	49	5.3	0.3	0.3	0
Salad dressing, blue cheese	1 tbsp.	77	8	0.7	1.1	0
Salad dressing, caesar	1 tbsp.	78	8.5	0.2	0.5	0
Salad dressing, coleslaw	1 tbsp.	61	5.2	0.1	3.7	0
Salad dressing, french	1 tbsp.	71	7	0.1	2.4	0
Salad dressing, honey dijon	1 tbsp.	57.5	5	0.5	3	0.5
Salad dressing, italian	1 tbsp.	43	4.2	0.1	1.5	0
Salad dressing, mayo-based	1 tbsp.	57	4.9	0.1	3.5	0
Salad dressing, mayonnaise	1 tbsp.	103	11.7	0	0	0
Salad dressing, peppercorn	1 tbsp.	76	8.2	0.2	0.5	0
Salad dressing, ranch	1 tbsp.	25	0	0	0	0
Salad dressing, russian	1 tbsp.	76	7.8	0.2	1.6	0
Salad, chicken	6 oz.	420	33	45	11	1.5
Salad, egg	6 oz.	300	23	20	14	0.5
Salad, prima pasta	6 oz.	360	30	4.8	18	2.5
Salad, seafood w/ crab & shrimp	6 oz.	420	34	0	20	0
Salad, tuna	6 oz.	450	36	16	14	0
Salami, cooked, turkey	1 oz.	37.7	2.3	0.7	0	0
Salami, dry, pork or beef	3 slices	104	8.1	6.3	1	0
Salami, italian pork	1 oz.	119	10.4	6.1	0.3	0
Salsa, w/ oil	2 tbsp.	40	3	0	8	0
Salsa, w/o oil	2 tbsp.	15	0	0	3.5	0
Salt	1 tbsp.	0	0	0	0	0
Sauce, alfredo	1/4 cup	120	11	15	3	2
Sauce, barbecue	1 cup	188	4.5	4.5	32	3
Sauce, cheese	1 cup	479	36.3	25.1	13.3	0.2
Sauce, cranberry	1 cup	418	0.4	0.6	107.8	2.8
Sauce, hollandaise	1 cup	62	1.5	2.3	10.3	0.2
Sauce, honey mustard	1 tbsp.	30	1	0	5	0
Sauce, marinara	1 cup	185	6	4.9	28.2	1
Sauce, salsa	1 cup	70	0.4	4	16.2	4.1
Sauce, soy	1 tbsp.	10	0	0	0	0
Sauce, steak	1 tbsp.	25	0	0	6	0
Sauce, teriyaki	1 tbsp.	15	0	17	2	0
Sauce, tomato chili	1 cup	284	0.8	6.8	54	16.1
Sauce, worcestershire	1 cup	184	0	0	53.5	0
Sauerkraut	1/2 cup	25	0	1	5	4
Sausage, italian pork, raw	1 link	391	35.4	16.1	0.7	0
Sausage, pork	1 link	85	7.4	4.2	0	0
Sausage, smoked linked, pork	1 link	265	21.6	15.1	1.4	0
Sausage, turkey	1 link	0	0	0	0	0
Savory, ground	1 tsp.	4	0.1	0.1	1	0.6
Scallops	1 scallop	26	0.2	5	0.7	0
Seaweed, dried	1 oz.	50	0	0	13	0
Sesame seeds, dried	1 tbsp.	52	4.5	1.6	2.1	1.1
Shallots	1 tbsp, chopped	7	0	0.3	1.7	0
Shortening	1 tbsp.	113	12.8	0	0	0
Shrimp, mixed species, raw	1 medium piece	6	0.1	1.2	0.1	0
Snacks, cheese puffs or twists	1 oz.	157	9.7	2.1	15.2	0.3

NUTRITIONAL INFORMATION

Nutrition values for fat, protein, carbohydrates, and fiber are listed in grams per serving.
Serving sizes and values are approximate.

FOOD ITEM	Serving Size	Cal.	Fat	Protein	Carbs	Fi
S (cont.)						
Soda, club	12 fl oz	0	0	0	0	0
Soda, cream	12 fl oz	252	0	0	65.7	0
Soda, diet cola	12 fl oz	0	0	0	0	0
Soda, ginger ale	12 fl oz	166	0	0	42.8	0
Soda, lemon-lime	12 fl oz	196	0	0	51.1	0
Soda, regular, w/ caffeine	12 fl oz	155	0	0.2	39.8	0
Soda, regular, w/o caffeine	12 fl oz	207	0	0.2	52.9	0
Soda, root beer	12 fl oz	202	0	0	52.3	0
Soda, tonic water	12 fl oz	166	0	0	42.9	0
Soup, beef broth	1 cup	29	0	5.3	1.7	0
Soup, beef stroganoff	1 cup	235	11	12.2	21.6	1
Soup, beef vegetable	1 cup	82	1.9	2.9	13.1	0
Soup, chicken broth	1 cup	39	1.3	4.9	0.9	0
Soup, chicken noodle	1 cup	75	2.4	4	9.3	0
Soup, chicken vegetable	1 cup	75	2.8	3.6	8.5	1
Soup, chicken w/ dumplings	1 cup	96	5.5	5.6	6	0
Soup, clam chowder	1 cup	95	2.8	4.8	12.4	0
Soup, cream of chicken	1 cup	117	7.3	3.4	9.2	0
Soup, cream of mushroom	1 cup	129	8.9	2.3	9.3	0
Soup, cream of potato	1 cup	149	6.4	5.7	17	0
Soup, minestrone	1 cup	82	2.5	4.2	11.2	1
Soup, split-pea w/ham	1 cup	190	4.4	10.3	27.9	2
Soup, tomato	1 cup	161	6	6.1	22.3	2
Soup, vegetarian	1 cup	72	1.9	2.1	11.9	0
Sour cream	1 tbsp	26	2.5	0.4	0.5	0
Sour cream, fat free	1 tbsp	9	0	0.3	1.8	0
Sour cream, reduced fat	1 tbsp	22	1.7	0.8	0.8	0
Soy milk	1 cup	127	4.7	10.9	12	3
Soy protein isolate	1 oz	96	1	22.9	2.1	1
Soybeans, green, cooked	1 cup	254	11.5	22.2	19.8	7
Soybeans, nuts, roasted	1/4 cup	194	9.2	17	14	3
Soyburger	1 patty	125	4.1	12.5	9.3	3
Spaghetti, cooked	1 cup	197	0.9	6.6	39.6	2
Spaghetti, spinach, cooked	1 cup	182	0.8	6.4	36.6	2
Spaghetti, whole-wheat, cooked	1 cup	174	0.7	7.4	37.1	6
Spinach	1 cup	7	0.1	0.9	1.1	0
Squab, boneless, raw	1 squab	585	47.4	36.8	0	0
Squab, skinless, raw	1 squab	239	12.6	29.4	0	0
Squash, summer	1 cup, sliced	18	0.2	1.4	3.8	1
Squash, winter	1 cup, cubed	39	0.2	1.1	10	1
Squid, mixed species, raw	1 oz	26	0.4	4.4	0.9	0
Stock, beef	1 cup	31	0.2	4.7	2.9	0
Stock, chicken	1 cup	86	2.9	6	8.5	0
Stock, fish	1 cup	40	1.9	5.3	0	0
Strawberries	1 cup	49	0.5	1	11.7	3
Succotash	1 piece	0	0	0	0	0
Sugar, brown	1 tsp	12	0	0	3.1	0
Sugar, granulated	1 tsp	16	0	0	4.2	0
Sugar, maple	1 tsp	11	0	0	2.7	0
Sugar, powdered	1 tsp	10	0	0	2.5	0

Nutrition values for fat, protein, carbohydrates, and fiber are listed in grams per serving.
Serving sizes and values are approximate.

FOOD ITEM	Serving Size	Cal.	Fat	Protein	Carbs	Fiber
S (cont.)						
Sunflower seeds	1 tbsp.	45	10	4	1.5	5
Sweet potato	1 cup, cubed	114	0.1	2.1	26.8	4
Syrup, chocolate	1 tbsp.	66.5	1.7	0.8	11.9	0.5
Syrup, dark corn	1 tbsp.	57	0	0	15.5	0
Syrup, grenadine	1 tbsp.	53	0	0	13.3	0
Syrup, light corn	1 tbsp.	59	0	0	15.9	0
Syrup, maple	1 tbsp.	52	0	0	13.4	0
Syrup, pancake	1 tbsp.	47	0	0	12.3	0.1
T						
Taco shell, hard	1 shell	55	3	2	6	0
Tangerines	1 large	52	0.3	0.8	13.1	1.8
Tarragon, dried	1 tsp.	2	0	0.1	0.3	0
Tea, instant	1 cup	2	0	0.1	0.4	0
Thyme	1 tsp.	1	0	0	0.2	0.1
Thyme, dried	1 tsp.	3	0.1	0.1	0.6	0.4
Tofu, firm	1/2 cup	183	11	19.9	5.4	2.9
Tofu, fried	1 piece	35	2.6	2.2	1.4	0.5
Tofu, soft	1/2 cup	75.5	4.6	8.1	2.2	0.2
Tomato juice, canned, with salt	6 fl oz.	31	0.1	1.4	7.7	0.7
Tomato juice, canned, without salt	6 fl oz.	30	0.1	1.2	7.8	0.7
Tomato paste, canned	1/2 cup	107	0.6	5.7	24.8	5.9
Tomato sauce, canned	1 cup	78	0.6	3.2	18.1	3.7
Tomatoes, canned, crushed	1 cup	82	0.7	4.2	18.6	4.8
Tomatoes, green	1 cup, chopped	41	0.4	2.2	9.2	2
Tomatoes, orange	1 cup, chopped	25	0.3	1.8	5	1.4
Tomatoes, red	1 cup, chopped	32	0.4	1.6	7.1	2.2
Tomatoes, sun-dried	1 cup, chopped	139	1.6	7.6	30.1	6.6
Toppings, butterscotch or caramel	2 tbsp.	103	0	0.6	27	0.4
Toppings, marshmallow cream	2 tbsp.	132	0.1	0.3	32.3	0
Toppings, nuts in syrup	2 tbsp.	184	9	1.8	23.8	0.9
Toppings, pineapple	2 tbsp.	106	0	0	27.9	0.2
Toppings, strawberry	2 tbsp.	107	0	0.1	27.8	0.3
Tortilla chips, plain	1 oz.	142	7.4	1.9	17.8	1.8
Tortilla, corn	1 tortilla	45	0.5	2	9	3
Tortilla, flour	1 tortilla	160	3	18	28	3
Trail mix	1/4 cup	173.2	11	5	16.8	3
Turkey, deli sliced, white meat	1 oz.	30	1	5	0.5	0
Turkey, back, skinless, boneless, raw	1/2 back	180	5.3	31	0	0
Turkey, breast, boneless, raw	1/2 breast	541	11.5	102.9	0	0
Turkey, breast, skinless, boneless, raw	1/2 breast	433	2.5	95.9	0	0
Turkey, dark meat, boneless, raw	1/2 turkey	686	25.5	106.7	0	0
Turkey, dark meat, skinless, boneless, raw	1/2 turkey	532	12.8	98	0	0
Turkey, leg, boneless, raw	1 leg	412	12.5	70.3	0	0
Turkey, leg, skinless, boneless, raw	1 leg	355	7.8	67	0	0
Turkey, wing, boneless, raw	1 wing	204	9.9	26.7	0	0
Turkey, wing, skinless, boneless, raw	1 wing	95	1	20.2	0	0
Turkey, young hen, back, boneless, raw	1/2 back	650	47.5	52.2	0	0
Turkey, young hen, breast, boneless, raw	1/2 breast	1460	72.5	189	0	0
Turkey, young hen, dark meat, boneless, raw	1/2 turkey	1056	39.6	163	0	0

NUTRITIONAL INFORMATION

Nutrition values for fat, protein, carbohydrates, and fiber are listed in grams per serving.
Serving sizes and values are approximate.

FOOD ITEM	Serving Size	Cal.	Fat	Protein	Carbs	Fi
T (cont.)						
Turkey, young hen, leg, boneless, raw	1 leg	991	49.2	127.7	0	0
Turkey, young hen, wing, boneless, raw	1 wing	470	31.1	44.6	0	0
Turkey, young tom, back, boneless, raw	1/2 back	938	58.4	96.8	0	0
Turkey, young tom, breast, boneless, raw	1/2 breast	2701	113.4	392.9	0	0
Turkey, young tom, dark meat, boneless, raw	1/2 turkey	1884	63	307	0	0
Turkey, young tom, leg, boneless, raw	1 leg	1740	78.2	241.1	0	0
Turkey, young tom, wing, boneless, raw	1 wing	654	39	71.2	0	0
Turnip greens	1 cup, chopped	18	0.2	0.8	3.9	1
Turnips	1 cup, cubed	36	0.1	1.2	8.4	2
V						
Vanilla extract	1 tbsp	37	0	0	1.6	0
Veal, breast, raw	1 oz	59	4.2	5	0	0
Veal, cubed, raw	1 oz	31	0.7	5.7	0	0
Veal, ground, raw	1 oz	41	1.9	5.5	0	0
Veal, leg, raw	1 oz	33	0.9	5.9	0	0
Veal, loin, raw	1 oz	46	2.6	5.4	0	0
Veal, rib, raw	1 oz	46	2.6	5.3	0	0
Veal, shank, raw	1 oz	32	1	5.4	0	0
Veal, shoulder, arm, raw	1 oz	37	1.5	5.5	0	0
Veal, shoulder, blade, raw	1 oz	37	1.5	5.5	0	0
Veal, shoulder, whole, raw	1 oz	37	1.5	5.5	0	0
Veal, sirloin, raw	1 oz	43	2.2	5.4	0	0
Vegetable juice	8 fl oz	50	0	2	12	2
Vinegar	1 tbsp	2	0	0	0.8	0
W						
Waffles, plain	1 waffle	218	10.6	5.9	24.7	0
Walnuts	1 oz. (14 halves)	185	18.5	4.3	3.9	1
Wasabi root	1 cup, sliced	142	0.8	6.2	30.6	1
Water chestnuts, chinese	1/2 cup, sliced	60	0.1	0.9	14.8	1
Watercress	1 cup, chopped	4	0	0.8	0.4	0
Watermelon	1 cup, diced	46	0.2	0.9	11.5	0
Wheat bran	1 cup	125	2.5	9	37.4	2
Wheat flour, whole grain	1 cup	407	2.2	16.4	87.1	1
Wheat germ	1 cup	414	11.2	26.6	59.6	1
Whipped cream	1 cup	154	13.3	1.9	7.5	0
Wine, cooking	1 tsp	2	0	0	0.3	0
Wine, red	3-1/2 oz. glass	74	0	0.2	1.8	0
Wine, rose	3-1/2 oz. glass	73	0	0.2	1.4	0
Wine, white	3-1/2 oz. glass	70	0	0.1	0.8	0
Yam	1 cup, cubed	177	0.3	2.3	41.8	6
Yeast, active, dry	1 tsp	12	0.2	1.5	1.5	0
Yogurt, fruit, low fat	8 oz. container	118	0.3	5.5	23.8	0
Yogurt, fruit, whole milk	8 oz. container	250	6	9	38	0
Yogurt, plain, lowfat	8 oz. container	110	4	7.9	7	0
Yogurt, plain, whole milk	8 oz. container	138	7.4	12	10.6	0
Z						
Zucchini	1 medium	45	0	2	10	1